CLINICAL
BACTERIOLOGY

J KEITH STRUTHERS
BSc (Hons), MSc, DPhil, MBChB, FRCPath
Consultant Medical Microbiologist
Coventry and Warwickshire Hospital
Coventry, UK

ROGER P WESTRAN
BSc, FIBMS
Senior Biomedical Scientist
Southend Hospital
Essex, UK

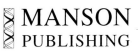
MANSON PUBLISHING

Acknowledgements

The authors wish to thank Brian Gee of the Coventry PHLS for his photographic skills.

Disclaimer

This book is written as a general education text for clinical bacteriology. In this setting, the organisms, clinical scenarios and diagnostic methods discussed relate to more common circumstances. In actual clinical practice other organisms may need to be considered.

Similarly, the information on antibiotics and antibiotic use in the text is for educational purposes. In the clinical setting, reference must be made to national documents such as the British National Formulary and local antibiotic guidelines, where contraindications, interactions and cautions are identified. The authors name specific agents as examples in a class of antibiotics for use in particular clinical settings. As such the authors do not have any commercial interest in a particular antibiotic. The statement in this paragraph also applies to vaccination, vaccines and diagnostic tests.

Second impression 2005

For full details of all Manson Publishing Ltd titles please write to:
Manson Publishing Ltd, 73 Corringham Road, London NW11 7DL, UK.
Tel: +44(0)20 8905 5150
Fax: +44(0)20 8201 9233
Website: www.mansonpublishing.com

Commissioning editor: Jill Northcott
Project manager: Paul Bennett
Colour reproduction: Acumen Colour Ltd
Printed by: Grafos SA, Barcelona, Spain

Contents

Preface

In the past many undergraduate medical school curricula were based on lecture-based courses in specific disciplines. Increasingly there has been a change to integrated problem-based teaching, with all the disciplines being integrated into a particular theme. While this has clear advantages, there are disadvantages as well. In the case of the pathologies, only a snapshot of a particular topic may be seen, and an overall understanding of a subject may be difficult for the student to obtain. Medical microbiology is one example of this, for in its own right it is a vast subject.

This book concentrates on bacteriology, and its aim is to provide a basic background for bacteriology and antibiotic use. Each chapter is written as an illustrated essay; there are four introductory chapters on bacteriology and antibiotic use, followed by nine based on the organ systems. Each of these chapters is divided into an introduction which covers aspects such as epidemiology, pathogenesis, diagnosis, treatment and public health issues. A comment section highlights other important issues. As with any part of medical microbiology, the science of bacteriology can be integrated with anatomy and histopathology, and aspects of this are highlighted in relevant sections. There are two final chapters on infections in the modern society and infection control.

We would thus see this book as providing the background to a particular problem-based clinical case, for example an older man with pulmonary tuberculosis or a young woman with pelvic inflammatory disease. Each relevant chapter provides an overview of the subject. Underpinning this is the basic theme of the book based on the gram stain feature of bacteria, and an introduction to the use of antibiotics centred on this simple feature of bacteria. This book has concentrated on common bacteria and conditions, and for the student who wishes to gain an insight into other organisms, there are many detailed and excellent texts.

Several specific examples of public health and antibiotic resistance issues in both the UK and the USA are given in the text. It is very important that the reader refers to the epidemiological data available for their own particular country, in order to appreciate the importance on these issues locally.

In addition to medical students, we consider the book has a wider audience, including doctors doing their specialist training, laboratory biomedical scientists, and nurses.

Keith Struthers
Roger Westran

Abbreviations

AAD antibiotic-associated diarrhoea
AFB acid-fast bacilli
AIDS acquired immunodeficiency syndrome
ALT alanine transaminase
APC antigen presenting cell
AST aspartate transaminase
ATP adenosine triphosphate
BCG Bacillus Calmette-Guerin
b.d. twice daily
BHI Brain Heart Infusion
BMS biomedical scientist
BSE bovine spongiform encephalopathy
BTS British Thoracic Society
cAb core antibody (of HBV)
cAg core antigen (of HBV)
cAMP cyclic adenosine monophosphate
CABG coronary artery bypass graft
CAP community acquired pneumonia
CAPD chronic ambulatory peritoneal dialysis
CCDC consultant in communicable disease control
CFT complement fixation test
CFTR cystic fibrosis transmembrane regulator
CMI cell-mediated immunity
CMV cytomegalovirus
COAD chronic obstructive airways disease
CPK creatinine phosphokinase
CRP C-reactive protein
CSF cerebrospinal fluid
CT computerized tomography
CTP cytidine triphosphate
CWM cold water mixer
CXR chest X-ray
DNA deoxyribonucleic acid
DNase deoxyribose nuclease
DOT directly observed therapy
DTH delayed type hypersensitivity
eAb e antibody (of HBV)
eAg e antigen (of HBV)
EBV Epstein Barr virus
EDTA ethylenediamine tetra-acetic acid
EEG electroencephalogram
EF (o)edema factor
EHO Environmental Health Officer
EIA enzyme immunoassay
ENT ear, nose, and throat
EPP exposure-prone procedure
ESBL extended spectrum β-lactamase
ESR erythrocyte sedimentation rate
ETT endotracheal tube
Factor X haemin
GABA γ-amino-n-butyric acid
GCU gonococcal urethritis
GISA glycopeptide intermediate *Staphylococcus aureus*
GP general practitioner
GUM genito-urinary medicine

HAP hospital acquired pneumonia
HAV hepatitis A virus
HBV hepatitis B virus
HCl hydrochloric acid
HCV hepatitis C virus
Hib *Haemophilus influenzae* type b
HBIG hepatitis B immunoglobulin
HIV human immunodeficiency virus
HPV human papilloma virus
HSV herpes simplex virus
ICC Infection control committee
ICD infection control doctor
ICN infection control nurse
ICT Infection control team
ICU intensive care unit
γ-IFN gamma interferon
Ig immunoglobulin
IG hyperimmune globulin
IL interleukin
INH isoniazid
i.v. intravenous
IVDU intravenous drug user
LF lethal factor
LFT liver function test
LJ Lowenstein Jensen
LP lumbar puncture
LRT lower respiratory tract
MBC minimum bactericidal concentration
MBL mannose binding lectin
MDR-TB multi-drug resistant tuberculosis
MHC major histocompatibility
MIC minimum inhibitory concentration
MMR measles, mumps, rubella
MRI magnetic resonance imaging
mRNA messenger RNA
MRSA methicillin resistant *Staphylococcus aureus*
MSSA methicillin sensitive *Staphylococcus aureus*
NAAT nucleic acid amplification test
NAD factor V (nicotinamide adenine dinucleotide)
NAG N-acetylglucosamine
NAM N-acetylmuramic acid
NGU non-gonococcal urethritis
NSAID non-steroidal anti-inflammatory drug
o.d. once daily
PA protective antigen
PBP penicillin binding protein
PCR polymerase chain reaction
PEP post-exposure prophylaxis
PID pelvic inflammatory disease
p.o. by mouth
PPD purified protein derivative
PrP polyribose-ribitol phosphate
PRP phospho-ribosyl pyrophosphate
PVE prosthetic valve endocarditis
PZA pyrazinamide

RBC red blood cell
RIF rifampicin
RNA ribonucleic acid
rRNA ribosomal ribonucleic acid
RSV respiratory syncitial virus
sAb surface antibody (of HBV)
sAg surface antigen (of HBV)
SIRS systemic inflammatory response syndrome
SRSV small round structured virus
STD sexually transmitted disease
STI sexually transmitted infection
TB tuberculosis
TCR T cell receptor
t.d.s. three times a day
Th T helper (cell)
TKR total knee replacement
TNF tumour necrosis factor

TORCHES toxoplasma, rubella, CMV, HSV, syphilis
TPHA *Treponema pallidum* haemagglutination
TPPA *Treponema pallidum* particle agglutination
tRNA transfer RNA
TSE transmissible spongiform encephalopathy
TSS toxic shock syndrome
U+E urea + electrolyte
UTI urinary tract infection
vCJD variant Creutzfeldt-Jakob disease
VDRL Venereal Disease Reference Laboratory
VRE vancomycin resistant enterococci
VZIG varicella zoster virus immunoglobulin
VZV varicella zoster virus
WBC white blood cell
WCC white cell count
ZN Ziehl-Neelsen

Normal Ranges and Conversion of Units

	SI units	*Traditional units*	*Conversion (SI to traditional)*
Haematology			
WCC			
Total	$4–10 \times 10^9/L$	$4–10 \times 10^3/mm^3$	
Neutrophils	$2–7.5 \times 10^9/L$	$2–7.5 \times 10^3/mm^3$	
CSF	$<5/\mu L$	$<5/mm^3$	
Urine	$<50/\mu L$	$<50/mm^3$	
Biochemistry			
ALT	5–30 iu/L	5–30 mu/mL	
Albumin	34–48 g/L	3.4–4.8 g/dL	$\div 10$
AST	10–40 iu/L	10–40 mu/mL	
Bilirubin	$2–17 \mu mol/L$	0.12–1.0 mg/dL	$\div 16.8$
C-reactive protein	0–10 mg/L	0–1.0 mg/dL	$\div 10$
Creatinine	$50–120 \mu mol/L$	0.57–1.36 mg/dL	$\times 0.0113$
Glucose	2.5–7.5 mmol/L	45–135 mg/dL	$\times 18.02$
Protein (CSF)	<0.45 g/L	<45 mg/dL	$\times 100$

UK and US Drug Names

UK drug name	US drug name
aciclovir	acyclovir
amoxycillin	amoxicillin
benzylpenicillin	penicillin G
cephazolin	cefazolin
clavulanic acid	clavulanate
co-amoxiclav	amoxicillin and clavulanate
co-trimoxazole	trimethoprim and sulfamethoxazole
rifampicin	rifampin

1 Structure and Function of Bacteria

Introduction

Most bacteria encountered in clinical practice are classified as gram-positive or gram-negative. As outlined below, this gram staining character is dependent on the structure of the bacterial cell wall. The stain enables determination of overall shape and size of an organism; bacteria are usually rod-like (bacillary), round (coccoid) or in the case of *Haemophilus influenzae*, cocco-bacillary (1).

The gram stain involves spreading a loop-full of specimen on a glass slide, which is then heat-fixed and subjected to various stains (2). Gram-positive bacteria retain the crystal violet/iodine complex and stain blue-black. With gram-negative bacteria, the crystal violet/iodine complex is eluted out when the outer lipid layer of the cell wall dissolves at the acetone step; they then take up the neutral red or safranine stain and appear pale red (3a, b). This simple technique is still central to diagnostic bacteriology, and has not been superseded by any modern molecular method. Within minutes of a specimen being processed in the laboratory, a gram stain result can be obtained. A gram stain of a specimen of cerebrospinal fluid

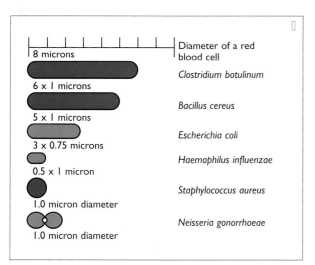

1 The size of selected bacteria in relation to the diameter of a red blood cell. Both gram-positive bacteria (blue) and gram-negative bacteria (red) can be bacillary, coccoid, or cocco-bacillary in shape.

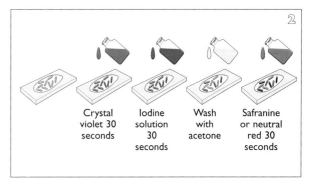

2 The gram stain procedure.

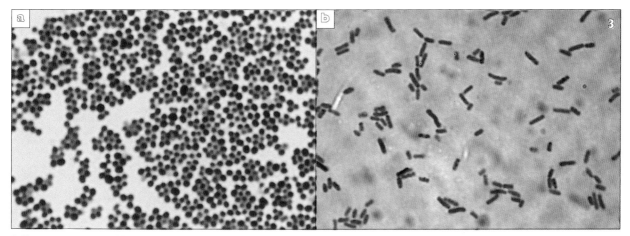

3 Photomicrographs of: (**a**) gram-positive cocci in clusters; (**b**) gram-negative rods.

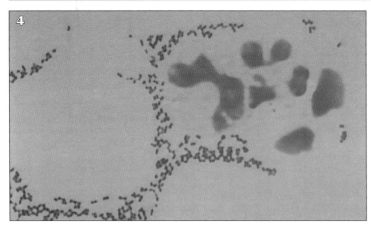

4 Photomicrograph of the CSF of a young child with the symptoms and signs of meningitis. Numerous gram-positive diplococci are seen around the red-stained nucleus of a neutrophil.

5 Common gram-positive, gram-negative and anaerobic bacteria encountered in clinical practice. Although flagella and capsules are usually not seen in the gram stain, they are indicated here and in subsequent diagrams for relevant bacteria.

(CSF) of a young child with meningitis shows numerous gram-positive diplococci scattered around a neutrophil (4). This child has pneumococcal meningitis.

Examples of bacteria to consider in many clinical situations are shown in 5. It is important to become familiar with these organisms, for in many circumstances the presumptive identification of the organism is made on the basis of the gram stain. In addition, the appropriateness of antibiotics being administered can also be assessed while the results of culture and susceptibility testing are awaited.

Certain bacteria are joined together in pairs (e.g. gonococcus, meningococcus and pneumococcus), in chains (e.g. streptococci and enterococci) or clusters (e.g. *Staphylococcus aureus* and the coagulase-negative staphylococci). These arrangements, seen in the gram stain, are also useful in making a presumptive identification of the organism in a specimen.

In addition to appreciating the importance of the gram stain, an understanding of the structure and function of the bacterial cell is important. Many aspects of structure and function are central to the pathogenic properties of individual bacteria. An outline of important components of a bacterial cell is shown in 6. As antibiotics target different sites of metabolism, it is relevant to have a basic understanding of the major macromolecular pathways such as DNA, RNA and protein synthesis.

Cell wall

The cell wall of a bacterium has many functions. The most important is to protect the inner cell structures from osmotic and other physical forces that a bacterium can encounter in a changing environment. Peptidoglycan is the major component of the gram-positive cell wall. In gram-negative bacteria, peptidoglycan lies between the cytoplasmic membrane and the outer lipid bilayer. The outer bilayer also contains lipopolysaccharide or endotoxin. A diagram showing features of the gram-positive and gram-negative cell wall is shown in 7.

The peptidoglycan polymer is cross-linked by side chains that consist of short peptides. These side chains are essential for the stability of the peptidoglycan and cell wall. Cross-linking is carried out by trans- and carboxy-peptidases, proteins anchored in the cytoplasmic membrane; these enzymes are also known as the penicillin binding proteins (PBP) (8). Note that while the number of

5

Organism	Gram stain features	Clinical importance – some examples
Aerobic/facultative bacteria		
Enterococci		Urinary tract infections, endocarditis
Streptococci A,B,C,D,G		A: pharyngitis, cellulitis B: neonatal sepsis
Viridans streptococci		Endocarditis, abscess, dental caries
Streptococcus pneumoniae		Community pneumonia, septic shock, meningitis
Staphylococcus aureus		Furunculosis, cellulitis, abscess, septic shock, endocarditis
Coagulase-negative staphylococci		Infection of prosthetic devices, bacteraemia
Escherichia coli		Urinary tract infections, septic shock, haemorrhagic colitis
Klebsiella spp.		Urinary tract infections, septic shock, pneumonia
Enterobacter/ citrobacter		Urinary tract infections, pneumonia, septic shock
Pseudomonas aeruginosa		Urinary tract infections, pneumonia, septic shock
Neisseria meningitidis		Septic shock, meningitis
Haemophilus influenzae		Respiratory tract infections
Anaerobes		
Clostridium spp.		Tetanus, botulism, infections of soft tissue, abdominal sepsis, abscess
Peptococcus/ Peptostreptococcus spp.		Infections of soft tissue, abdominal sepsis, abscess
Bacteroides/Porphyromonas/Prevotella spp.		Infections of soft tissue, abdominal sepsis, abscess

6 The outline of a bacterial cell showing important structural and functional components. (DNA: deoxyribonucleic acid; RNA: ribonucleic acid; mRNA: messenger RNA; tRNA: transfer RNA; rRNA: ribosomal RNA.)

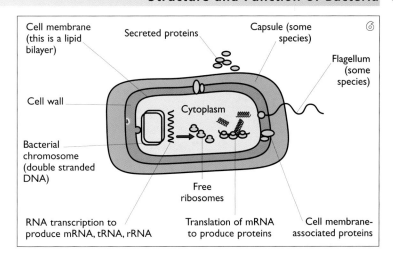

6 The outline of a bacterial cell showing important structural and functional components.

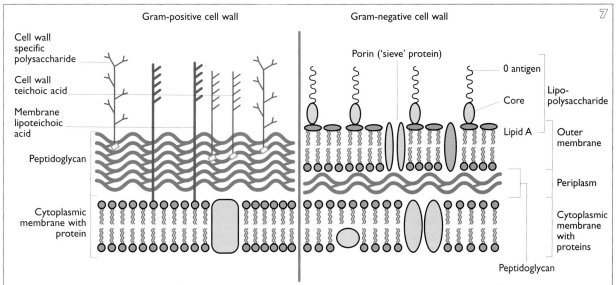

7 The structure of the cell wall of gram-positive and gram-negative bacteria.

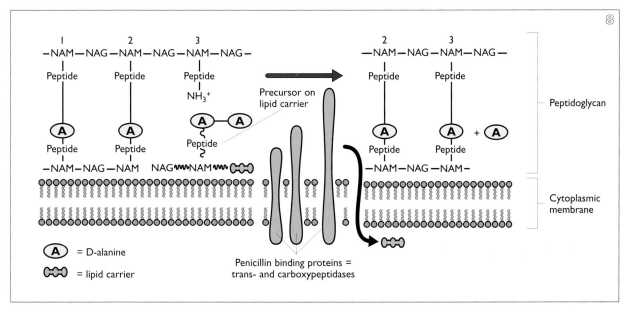

8 Peptidoglycan consists of repeating units of N-acetylglucosamine (NAG) and N-acetylmuramic acid (NAM) cross-linked by peptide side chains. The penicillin binding proteins (PBP) are responsible for cross-linking these peptide side chains.

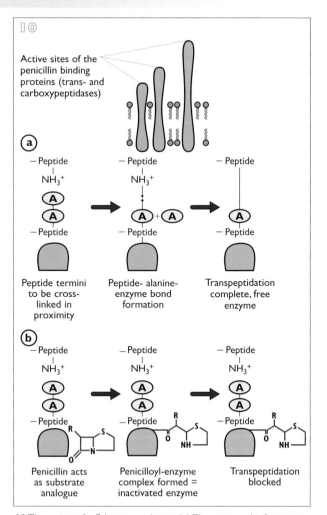

9 An outline of the structure of β-lactam antibiotics. The arrow shows the bond in the β-lactam ring that accounts for the antimicrobial activity of the β-lactam antibiotics.

different PBP may be five or more, three are used for illustrative purposes in this book. These proteins are the sites of action of the β-lactam antibiotics (penicillins, cephalosporins, and carbapenems) whose activity resides in the β-lactam ring (**9**). Covalent binding of a β-lactam agent to the active site of a PBP inactivates the enzyme, preventing cross-linking of the peptidoglycan polymers (**10a, b**); the consequence is cell death.

The cell wall of gram-negative bacteria is more complex than that of gram-positive bacteria (**7**). The outer lipid bilayer has proteins, such as adhesins and flagella traversing this membrane. The porins act as ion channels to allow hydrated molecules to pass through the membrane. From the periplasmic space, molecules can be transported across the cytoplasmic membrane into the cell. It should be noted that these porins enable antibiotics such as the β-lactams to reach their site of action. Benzylpenicillin is not effective against most gram-negative organisms because it is not sufficiently polar to pass through a porin channel. Ampicillin, a commercial derivative of benzylpenicillin, differs in the addition of an amino group on the side chain (**11**). Ampicillin is sufficiently polar for it to pass through the hydrated porin channel into the periplasmic space where it can act on the PBP.

Bacterial physiology

Bacteria function by many complex and interacting biochemical pathways. Energy to drive these pathways needs to be provided by a carbon source such as glucose. Physiologically, bacteria are classed as aerobic, where oxygen is essential for growth (e.g. *Pseudomonas aeruginosa*); facultative, where the organism can grow in the presence or absence of oxygen (e.g. the gram-negative 'coliforms'); and anaerobic, where the bacteria have to grow in the absence of oxygen (e.g. clostridia and bacteroides).

10 The action of a β-lactam antibiotic. (**a**) The steps in the formation of the peptide cross-link of the peptidoglycan chain. (**b**) β-lactam antibiotics bind covalently to the active site of the penicillin binding proteins preventing the transpeptidation step, and the cross-link is not formed.

11 The structure of (**a**) benzylpenicillin and (**b**) ampicillin.

When obligate aerobic bacteria such as *Pseudomonas aeruginosa* and facultative 'coliforms' grow in oxygen, glucose is completely metabolized by aerobic respiration, using oxygen as the final electron acceptor:

$$\text{Glucose} + 6O_2 \rightarrow 6H_2O + 6CO_2 \quad \Delta G^o = -686 \text{ kcal/mole}$$

When 'coliforms' grow in the absence of oxygen, they metabolize glucose by the less efficient process of fermentation, where mixed acids are the end products. This reaction is as follows:

$$2\text{Glucose} + H_2O \rightarrow 2\text{lactate} + \text{acetate} + \text{ethanol} + 2CO_2 + 2H_2$$

$$\Delta G^o = -47 \text{ kcal/mole}$$

Note that the amount of energy produced from a mole of glucose by aerobic respiration is much greater than that produced by fermentation.

The mode of metabolism that facultative organisms such as 'coliforms' are in at a particular time influences the action of some antibiotics. The aminoglycosides, such as gentamicin, act on 'coliforms' that are growing in the presence of oxygen, because these antibiotics probably enter the cell by an energy dependent process which is part of aerobic respiration.

Organisms such as streptococci and enterococci can grow in the presence or absence of oxygen, but they always use fermentation. For anaerobic bacteria, molecular oxygen derivatives such as superoxide are toxic; these organisms do not have the necessary enzyme systems to inactivate these toxic radicals, hence they grow only in the absence of oxygen.

From a practical laboratory aspect, the different requirements of bacteria for oxygen are important. The correct gaseous conditions must be available to ensure that obligate aerobes, facultative organisms, or obligate anaerobes are isolated from clinical specimens. For the routine culture of anaerobic bacteria from clinical specimens, all laboratories must have an anaerobic cabinet, or similar system, from which oxygen is excluded.

Synthesis of DNA, RNA and proteins

The bacterial genome consists of double-stranded DNA approximately 1,000 microns (1 mm) in length and replication occurs in a semi-conservative fashion. DNA replication produces two 'daughter' genomes, then the 'mother' cell divides to produce two 'daughter' cells. The daughters divide giving rise to exponential growth (**12a, b**). Most bacteria divide every 20 minutes or so under optimum growth conditions, hence a single organism inoculated onto an agar plate will have reproduced to form a visible colony the next day. In contrast, *Mycobacterium tuberculosis* divides every 18 hours or so, and under standard laboratory conditions it can take several weeks for a colony to be seen. With semi-

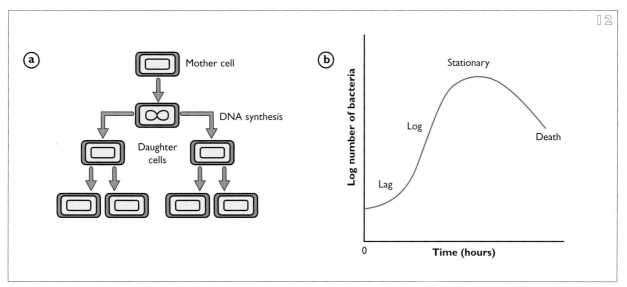

12 (**a**) Replication and cell division give rise to logarithmic growth, where bacteria divide into 2, 4, 8 organisms and so on. (**b**) A growth curve; when nutrients and other factors become self-limiting, the bacterial population enters a stationary and then death phase.

conservative replication the two parent strands separate and daughter DNA is laid down (**13a, b**); a DNA polymerase enzyme complex is responsible for this (**13c**). Details of the action of this enzyme complex at the molecular level are shown in **13d**.

The genome of an organism such as *Escherichia coli* has a length of about 1000 microns and has to fit into a cell 3 × 1 microns. To accomplish this, the genome has to be supercoiled (**14a**). This involves the topoisomerase enzymes, which include DNA gyrase whose mode of action is shown in **14b**. An important group of antibiotics, the fluorinated quinolones (e.g. ciprofloxacin and norfloxacin), bind to the α-subunit and inactivate the enzyme.

DNA is divided into sequences of nucleotides that code for proteins via messenger RNA (mRNA). These sequences are arranged into transcription units termed operons. An operon consists of a promotor/operator region, a region that codes for the protein, and a 'termination' region (**15a**). The RNA polymerase complex carries out the transcription of mRNA from the DNA chromosome (**15b**). The action of this enzyme is inhibited by the antibiotic rifampicin (RIF).

The regulation of gene expression at the transcription level is central in coordinating the metabolic activity of the cell. In procaryotic organisms such as bacteria, it is usual for all the enzymes necessary for a particular metabolic pathway to be expressed by means of one polycistronic mRNA molecule. The pattern of expression of the lactose operon of *Escherichia coli*, which codes for three enzymes, β-galactosidase, permease, and trans-acetylase, is shown in **16**. All three enzymes are needed for uptake into the cell and initial processing of the carbohydrate lactose.

Protein synthesis

Ribosomes translate mRNA molecules to produce proteins. Each three nucleotide 'codon' of the mRNA specifies a particular amino acid. All protein synthesis starts with the amino acid formylmethionine, coded by the sequence AUG, the initiation codon. An outline of protein synthesis is shown in **17**. Two ribosomal subunits bind specifically to one end of mRNA. Individual ribosomes move down the mRNA molecule, and as each three base codon is 'read', an amino acid is inserted into the growing peptide chain. At the end of each coding sequence on the mRNA, 'stop' codons such as UAA specify chain termination, and the completed peptide chain is released. The ribosomal subunits recycle to form new initiation complexes. The process of translation is the target of a number of important antibiotics.

Cytoplasmic membrane and some of its functions

Eucaryotic cells have several lipid bilayer membrane systems where they can organize metabolic and synthetic functions. These include the mitochondrial, nuclear, and cytoplasmic membranes, the endoplasmic reticulum, and the Golgi apparatus. Bacteria have only one membrane system, the cytoplasmic membrane, which delimits the cytoplasm from the cell wall. This membrane is essential

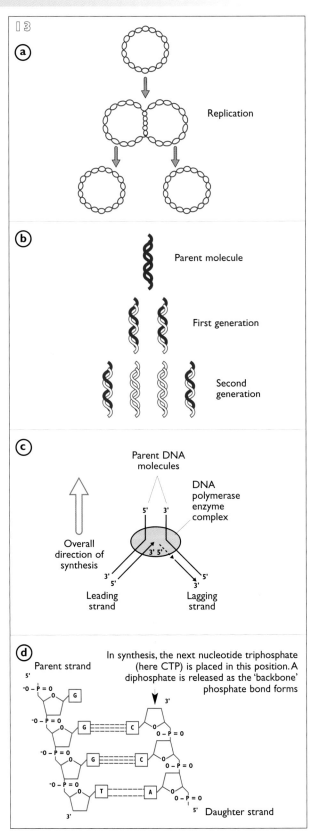

13 (**a**) One bacterial genome replicates to produce two 'daughters'. (**b**) The 'mother' deoxyribonucleic acid (DNA) strands separate and a 'daughter' strand is laid down. (**c**) An outline of the DNA polymerase complex. (**d**) Synthesis of a daughter strand relies on specific 'base pairing'. (CTP: cytidine triphosphate.)

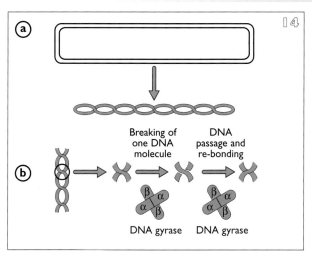

14 (a) The deoxyribonucleic acid (DNA) chromosome has to be supercoiled to fit into a cell. (b) Strand breakage and crossover are essential in this process, which is performed by enzymes such as DNA gyrase.

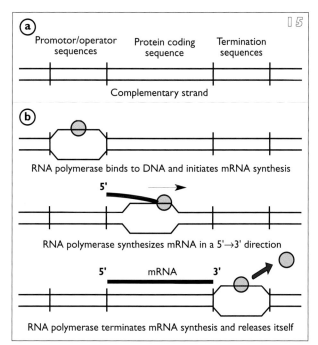

15 (a) DNA is divided into sequences that code for particular proteins. There are 'promotor/operator' and 'termination' sequences at the beginning and end of every transcription complex. (b) An outline of the process of transcription.

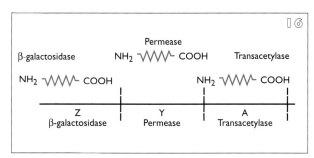

16 The organization of the lactose operon of *Escherichia coli*.

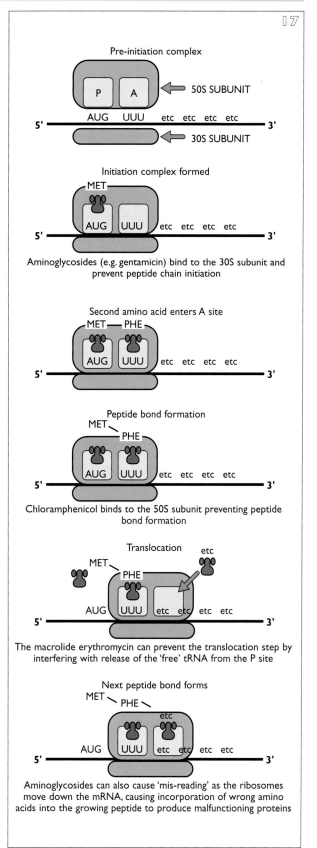

17 An outline of protein synthesis. Many antibiotics interfere with protein synthesis. (P: peptidyl; A: acceptor site of the 50S subunit; MET: formylmethionine; PHE: phenylalanine, the codon for which is UUU.)

for the transport of a wide range of compounds both in and out of the cell. Metabolic and structural entities reside in the cytoplasmic membrane, which has the basic structure of all lipid bilayers (7).

Protein synthesis

Proteins that are destined to reside in the cytoplasmic membrane or that are to be secreted out of the cell are synthesized in the proximity of the cytoplasmic membrane (18). Specific sequences at the amino terminal end of the growing peptide chain enable the protein to enter the cytoplasmic membrane. A protein may be completely secreted, as occurs with the enterotoxin of *Vibrio cholerae*, or it can be anchored in the cytoplasmic membrane where it will have a specific function. The proteins making up the electron transport chain of 'oxidative' gram-negative bacteria and the PBP are examples of anchored proteins. Other important protein structures resident in the cytoplasmic membrane are adhesins and flagella.

Adhesin proteins

An essential pathogenic property of many bacteria is the ability to adhere to epithelial and endothelial surfaces. Adhesin proteins enable this to occur. Uropathogenic strains of *Escherichia coli*, commonly associated with urinary tract infections (UTI), colonize the periurethral area of susceptible females by specific adhesins, which recognize receptors on the host cell surface (19). From here the bacteria gain access to the bladder via the urethra and initiate cystitis.

Flagellum

Many bacteria are motile and this is due to the presence of one or more flagella. Examples of flagellated bacteria include *Escherichia coli*, *Vibrio cholerae*, and *Clostridium tetani*. Flagella are complex protein structures anchored in the cell membrane. In conjunction with chemical signalling systems, bacteria can use their flagella to move towards a source of nutrients or away from an unfavourable environment. The basic structure of a flagellum is shown in 20. Flagella can occur all over the cell, as in coliforms (peritrichous), or they can be restricted to one end as found with *Pseudomonas aeruginosa*.

Capsules

The capsule is a structure exterior to the cell wall. A number of gram-positive and gram-negative bacteria are encapsulated. Capsules, usually consisting of a poly-saccharide, enable the bacterium to resist phagocytosis by macrophages and neutrophils (21). In fact, injection of millions of unencapsulated pneumococci into the peritoneum of a mouse is not lethal, while injecting a few hundred encapsulated organisms is.

Examples of important encapsulated bacteria, their various capsular serotypes, and available vaccines are shown in 22. Development of an immune response to specific capsular material can give protection against an organism. Clinically, the most important serotype of *Haemophilus influenzae* is serotype b (Hib), which can cause invasive disease such as bacteraemia, meningitis, and epiglottitis in

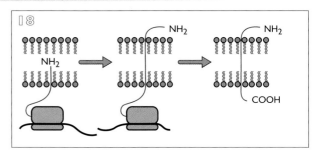

18 The cytoplasmic membrane has the typical lipid bilayer structure. Proteins such as the penicillin binding protein are synthesized on ribosomes adjacent to the membrane.

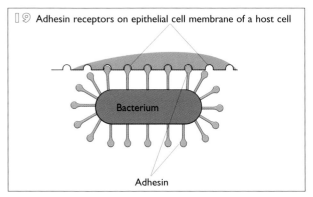

19 Adhesin proteins enable bacteria to adhere to specific receptors on the surface of host cells.

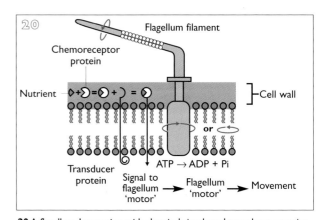

20 A flagellum. Interaction with chemical signals and transducer proteins determines which direction the flagellum and the bacterium moves. (ADP; adenosine diphosphate; ATP: adenosine triphosphate.)

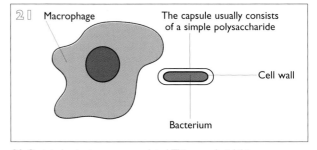

21 Certain bacteria are encapsulated. This capsule inhibits phagocytosis and is an important pathogenic property of bacteria such as *Haemophilus influenzae*, pneumococcus and meningococcus.

	Organism	Capsule type	Vaccine
	Haemophilus influenzae	6: a,b,c,d,e,f	Hib (polysaccharide of capsule serotype b conjugated to a carrier protein)
	Neisseria meningitidis	8: A,B,C,X,Y, Z,E,W-135	A,C,Y,W-135 (B capsular material is non-immunogenic)
	Streptococcus pneumoniae	>90: e.g. 3,10, 19	23 common serotypes in the single vaccine

22 Three important encapsulated bacteria, with the number and classification of the serotypes and available vaccines indicated. (Hib: *Haemophilus influenzae* type b.)

children less than 5 years old. Disease due to serotype b is now rare in countries where Hib vaccination is practised.

The Hib vaccine is an example of the outstanding success that an effective vaccine has on public health. The purified capsule polysaccharide (polyribose-ribitol phosphate; PrP) of Hib is antigenic when bound to a carrier protein. The Hib vaccine thus consists of PrP bound to a protein such as the tetanus toxoid. Antibodies are produced to the PrP component as well as to the tetanus toxoid. The antibodies produced to the PrP are protective and any invading haemophilus of serotype b will bind the antibodies produced as a result of vaccination. The function of the capsule is thus neutralized, enabling phagocytosis of the bacterium and its subsequent destruction.

Sporulation

Medically important bacteria including *Clostridium botulinum*, *Clostridium tetani*, and *Bacillus cereus* produce spores. Under unfavourable growth conditions the vegetative cell produces a heat stable spore (**23**). These spores can survive for years. When growth conditions are favourable, the spores germinate and vegetative growth is re-established. In a clinical setting it is bacteria that may have survived in soil or in cooked food as spores which then germinate. The resulting population of vegetative bacteria produces the toxins that are directly responsible for the disease.

Genetic exchange in bacteria

DNA can be transferred between bacteria by bacterial viruses (bacteriophages), by transformation, or by conjugation. Many bacteria contain extra-chromosomal plasmids which can occur as one or more copies per cell (**24a**). If there are two or more copies per cell, each daughter cell will usually inherit a plasmid after cell division. Plasmids can also transfer from a 'male' F$^+$ cell to a 'female' F$^-$ cell by the process of conjugation (**24b**). In this process the 'male' cell remains 'male'. Plasmids can thus be spread vertically from one generation to the next at cell division, or horizontally by the process of conjugation.

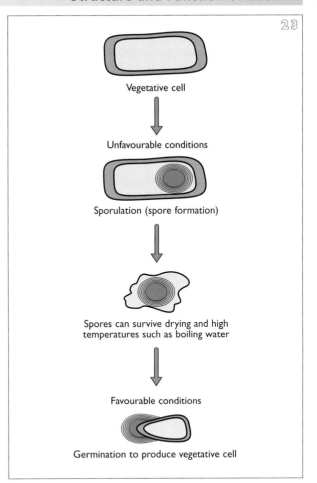

Vegetative cell

Unfavourable conditions

Sporulation (spore formation)

Spores can survive drying and high temperatures such as boiling water

Favourable conditions

Germination to produce vegetative cell

23 Bacteria such as clostridia and bacillus sporulate under unfavourable growth conditions.

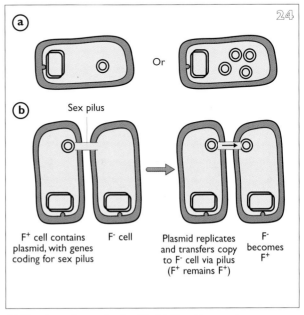

(a)

Or

(b) Sex pilus

F$^+$ cell contains plasmid, with genes coding for sex pilus   F$^-$ cell   Plasmid replicates and transfers copy to F$^-$ cell via pilus (F$^+$ remains F$^+$)   F$^-$ becomes F$^+$

24 Many bacteria contain plasmids. (**a**) Plasmids can exist as one or more copies per cell. (**b**) Plasmids can transfer between bacteria by the process of conjugation. A sex pilus, a simple protein tube, is necessary for this process.

As many plasmids carry genes coding for antibiotic resistance, the spread of plasmids is central to the problem of antibiotic resistance. A common form of resistance in the gram-negative Enterobacteriaceae, or 'coliforms', is the production of β-lactamase enzyme that hydrolyses the β-lactam ring of antibiotics such as benzylpenicillin, ampicillin, and amoxycillin. Often the resistance gene is carried on a plasmid; an example is the gene coding for the TEM-1 β-lactamase, which is widespread amongst the 'coliforms'.

Comment

This chapter provides a brief overview of the structure and function of bacteria. All aspects of these topics are important in understanding the pathogenic properties of bacteria, the action of antibiotics, and antibiotic resistance mechanisms. There are many excellent textbooks on the science of microbiology and the student who is interested should browse through these books in the medical school library.

From a practical aspect in medical education, it is an understanding of gram stain and an appreciation of basic properties of bacteria that is important. When doing clinical teaching sessions on the ward it is worthwhile to note any gram stain results, such as those found with positive blood cultures. These results should be followed up on subsequent days, when the identity and antibiotic sensitivity profile of the organism are available, to determine how the patient is managed.

One of the most exciting areas of research in the biological sciences in the last half of the twentieth century was in the area of bacterial genetics and virology. The study of plasmids, transposons and bacteriophages, combined with the development of methods to sequence DNA and RNA, have provided the methodology to manipulate the genetic makeup of any living organism. In addition, this research is the basis of modern diagnostic techniques such as the polymerase chain reaction (PCR). Modern textbooks provide a useful introduction to these topics.

It is interesting to investigate in more detail the differences between procaryotic organisms such as bacteria and the more 'complex' eucaryotes. One major difference is the process of transcription. In eucaryotes, genes specifying a protein are divided into coding sequences termed exons, which are separated from each other by non-coding introns. All the exons and introns appear in the mRNA that is transcribed. The introns are then spliced out of the RNA to produce the mRNA coding for a single protein. It is fascinating to examine the replication of the human immunodeficiency virus (HIV), as this virus has to parasitize the splicing mechanism of the eucaryotic cell in order to reproduce.

2 How Bacteria Cause Disease

Introduction

There are a number of ways that bacteria can cause disease. Pharyngitis and vaginitis are examples of infections occurring on epithelial surfaces. In addition to these superficial infections, bacteria can cause disease by invasion of a site usually considered to be sterile, such as the bladder or the blood. When *Streptococcus pneumoniae* enters the blood, it is distributed throughout the body, and can invade other organs including the brain and heart, causing meningitis and endocarditis respectively.

Botulism, tetanus, and cholera are toxin-mediated conditions. A growing population of bacteria produce extracellular proteins, or exotoxins, and it is these toxins that directly cause the disease.

Other diseases have an immunological basis. For example, Guillain-Barré syndrome, a progressive but usually reversible polyneuropathy, may develop following gastroenteritis caused by campylobacter. Here the immune response to the organism initiates an inflammatory reaction affecting the myelin sheath and the axon of nerves, giving rise to the polyneuropathy. Acute rheumatic fever also has an immunological basis. Antibodies produced to the surface M protein of group A streptococcus cross-react with certain host proteins, the most important being in the heart, and the heart valves in particular. The inflammatory response arising from this process leads to fibrosed and damaged valves.

Defences of the body

The major defences of the body against micro-organisms can be divided into non-specific or active, the latter based on the immune response. Some examples of defences are shown in **25**.

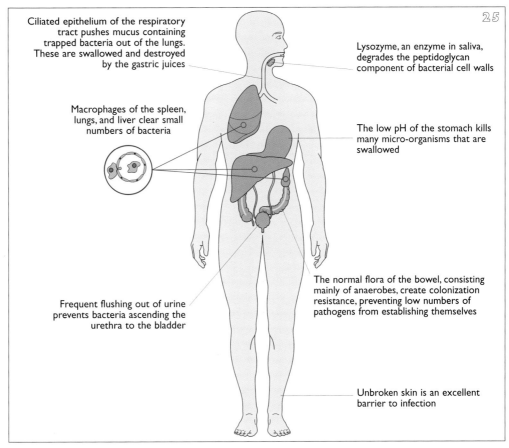

25 Some examples of anatomical, physiological, immune-based and microbial defences of the body.

Ciliated epithelium of the respiratory tract pushes mucus containing trapped bacteria out of the lungs. These are swallowed and destroyed by the gastric juices

Lysozyme, an enzyme in saliva, degrades the peptidoglycan component of bacterial cell walls

Macrophages of the spleen, lungs, and liver clear small numbers of bacteria

The low pH of the stomach kills many micro-organisms that are swallowed

Frequent flushing out of urine prevents bacteria ascending the urethra to the bladder

The normal flora of the bowel, consisting mainly of anaerobes, create colonization resistance, preventing low numbers of pathogens from establishing themselves

Unbroken skin is an excellent barrier to infection

Non-specific defences

These defences may be classified as anatomical, physiological and bacteriological. The intact skin is a barrier to infection and a surgical or traumatic incision will compromise the integrity of the skin; post-operative wound infections are a problem in surgery. Microanatomical defences are also important. The ciliated epithelium of the respiratory tract is responsible for pushing the mucus produced by goblet cells out of the lungs. Bacteria trapped in the mucus are prevented from entering the sterile parts of the respiratory tract such as the alveoli. In smokers it is recognized that the action of the mucociliary epithelium of the respiratory tract is compromised by the toxic effect of smoke. Otherwise healthy immunocompetent smokers are more likely to develop pneumococcal pneumonia than their non-smoking counterparts.

Physiological defences are found in the stomach and the bladder. The normal acidic environment of the stomach will kill many organisms that are swallowed. The bladder can be regarded as being sterile, but in the female in particular it is reasonable to assume that small numbers of bacteria enter the bladder via the urethra. The flushing out of the urine at micturition usually prevents these bacteria from establishing a nidus of infection.

Micro-organisms themselves constitute a defence system of the body. It is important to appreciate that humans have a normal bacterial flora on the skin and the mucous membranes such as the nasopharynx. Most of these bacteria are commensals. The bacterial flora of the colon contributes to the normal physiology of the colon and bacteria make up about 30% of the dry weight of faeces. About 99.9% of this bacterial flora is anaerobes, which include *Bacteroides* spp. and *Peptostreptococcus* spp. If the composition of this normal flora is altered, for example by broad-spectrum antibiotics, pathogens such as toxin-producing *Clostridium difficile* can overgrow, resulting in antibiotic-associated diarrhoea.

Active defences

The active defence system is based on the immune response. This system must be the most complex found in living organisms, and it has been central to the development and survival of higher animals. It is based on the ability of higher animals to differentiate self from non-self, and thus identify and destroy invading micro-organisms. Infectious diseases are largely concerned with organisms that are true pathogens for the immunocompetent individual. However, the true magnificence of the immune system to ward off all types of organisms is revealed when infection in immunocompromised individuals is considered. Acquired immunodeficiency syndrome (AIDS) in the patient infected with HIV is the classic example. Here organisms that generally do not cause infection in immunocompetent individuals do so in the AIDS patient. The same applies to the leukaemic or organ transplant patient who is on immunosuppressive drugs.

What stimulates the immune response against an invading pathogen? The key cells at the start of the process are the phagocytic cells such as the tissue macrophages, which have the ability to take up micro-organisms and destroy them. The first step is uptake of the organism into a phagosome. The latter fuses with another cytoplasmic vesicle, the

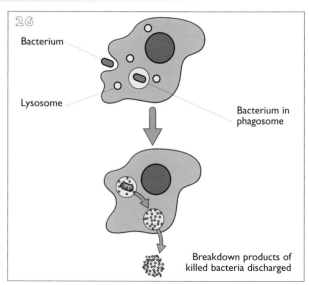

26 A phagocytic cell takes up a bacterium into a phagosome; fusion with the lysosome enables the organism to be killed.

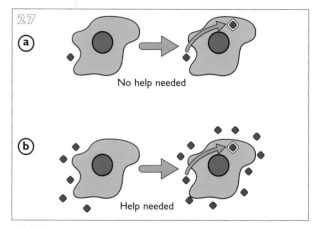

27 (**a**) A macrophage may be able to take up one pathogen and destroy it. (**b**) Large numbers of the pathogen will overwhelm the macrophage and it has to recruit help.

lysosome, containing oxygen radicals, acid hydrolases, peroxidases, and lysozymes responsible for destruction of the organism. The final breakdown products of the organism are then ejected from the cell (**26**).

If a few organisms enter a sterile site in the body such as an alveolus, the resident macrophages will take them up and destroy them; if large numbers of the organism enter the same site the resident macrophages may be overwhelmed (**27a, b**). The macrophages must signal their plight promptly to other cells of the immune system, and the T lymphocyte is the key in this process. The consequence of a successful outcome, where the infection is controlled, is that other macrophages and neutrophils are brought to the site of the infection; their phagocytic and destructive properties are enhanced and the infection is aborted. A number of different cell types, cytokine and chemokine protein signals, and antibodies, are all integral parts of this response. Some features of the main cells involved are shown in **28**.

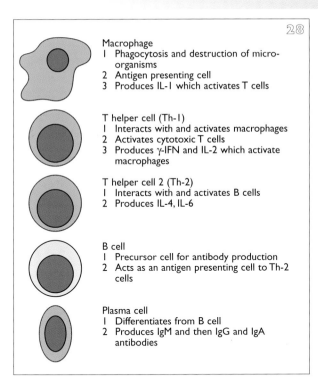

Macrophage
1 Phagocytosis and destruction of micro-organisms
2 Antigen presenting cell
3 Produces IL-1 which activates T cells

T helper cell (Th-1)
1 Interacts with and activates macrophages
2 Activates cytotoxic T cells
3 Produces γ-IFN and IL-2 which activate macrophages

T helper cell 2 (Th-2)
1 Interacts with and activates B cells
2 Produces IL-4, IL-6

B cell
1 Precursor cell for antibody production
2 Acts as an antigen presenting cell to Th-2 cells

Plasma cell
1 Differentiates from B cell
2 Produces IgM and then IgG and IgA antibodies

28 Some important cells of the immune response. (IFN: interferon; Ig: immunoglobulin; IL: interleukin.)

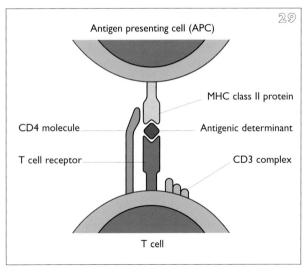

29 The macrophage presents antigen ♦ with the MHC-II proteins. This specific structure is recognized by one set of T cells only. Proteins such as CD4 and CD3 are essential in enhancing this specificity. (MHC: major histocompatibility.)

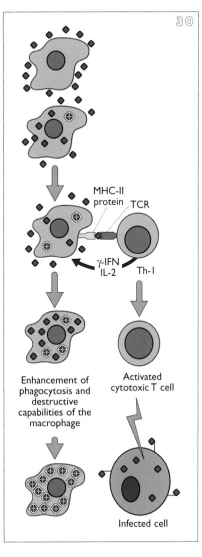

30 A macrophage takes up ♦ and presents it with the MHC-II protein. This is recognized by the T cell receptor of a specific population of Th-1 cells. γ-IFN and IL-2 from the T cell stimulate the macrophage to take up more ♦ and destroy it. Cytotoxic T cells, which recognize ♦ with the MHC-I protein on other cells, are also activated to destroy these cells.

The macrophage takes up foreign material (an antigen) with the aim of destroying it. Such cells are also antigen-presenting cells (APC) and present a small part of an antigen, the antigenic determinant, on the cell surface. It is here that the specificity of the immune response is initiated. The antigenic determinant, with its unique structure, is presented in the arms of the major histocompatibility type II (MHC-II) proteins on the surface of the APC. The MHC-II proteins are restricted to cells of the immune system, in contrast to the MHC-I proteins that are widely distributed amongst all other cells of the body.

There are small populations of T lymphocytes in every individual, specific for every conceivable foreign antigenic determinant that an individual may come in contact with during his or her life. An APC such as a macrophage with a unique antigenic determinant on its surface will be recognized by the population of T cells that have T cell receptors (TCRs) specific for that complex (**29**). If an organism has a number of antigenic determinants, for example ●♠♦♥, these four different determinants would each be recognized by four different sets of T cells, each waiting for that specific determinant to be presented to them by an APC.

For the purposes of this section consider that the 'organism' is an antigen consisting of a single antigenic determinant ♦. In order to recognize and mount an effective response against ♦, several cell types are involved. Macrophages initiate one part of the response, and after taking up ♦ and attempting to destroy it, also present ♦ to the T helper cells (Th-1). These T cells proliferate and activate, via gamma interferon (γ-IFN) and interleukin-2 (IL-2), the macrophages so that they can effectively destroy ♦ (**30**).

In addition the Th-1 cells activate cytotoxic T cells to search out any cells in the body that may be expressing ♦ on their surface and kill them. This applies in particular to virus-infected cells that usually express viral antigens on their surfaces (**30**). In these virus-infected cells which are not part of the immune system, the antigen appears on the surface with the MHC-I protein. It is here that the immune system is able to recognize cells that are infected, and differentiate them from immune system cells such as macrophages that express the antigen with the MHC-II protein. The stimulated cytotoxic T cell is the basis of cell-mediated immunity (CMI).

The other arm of the immune response results in antibody production, and is initiated by the B lymphocyte. In each individual there is a small population of B cells specific for every conceivable antigenic determinant, such as ♦, the example used here. These B cells have on their surfaces IgM and IgD antibodies which act as receptors specific for that determinant. Acting as APC, they recognize ♦ and bind it via the immunglobulin receptors, internalize and then present ♦ to Th-2 cells in the presence of the MHC-II proteins. Cytokines, including IL-4 and IL-6, activate the B cell, which matures into a plasma cell that synthesizes antibodies that are specific for ♦

(**31**). After several days, IgM and then IgG and IgA antibodies are released by the plasma cells (**32a**). They will bind to antigen ♦ and in this bound form the antigen is 'neutralized' (**32b**). Antigen bound to antibody is more readily phagocytosed by macrophages and neutrophils.

Following a successful response to a foreign antigen, populations of T and B memory cells for that antigen are maintained. They can mount an immediate response when the individual is exposed to the antigen in the future. This is the basis of vaccination.

Acute reaction to infection

The problem with the antibody response is that antibodies start to appear 4–5 days after the immune system recognizes an organism as foreign. In the case of meningococcal or pneumococcal infection this antibody response will be too late in helping to overcome the acute infection. Within a matter of hours, the infected person may either recover with no medical intervention, recover because antibiotics are given promptly, or die. Other arms of the immune defence are of critical importance in fighting an infection in the early stages. The interaction of the macrophage with the T cell initiates the

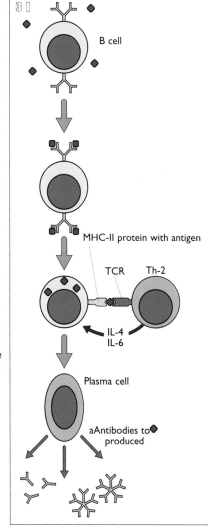

31 B cells with immunoglobulin receptors recognize ♦ which is presented on the surface with the MHC-II proteins. This is recognized by the T cell receptor of a specific population of Th-2 cells. IL-4 and IL-6 activate the B cell to mature into an antibody producing plasma cell.

32 (a) Antibodies are released from plasma cells after a number of days. Pentameric IgM is produced first, followed by a switch to IgG and IgA. **(b)** The specific antigenic determinant (♦) binds to the Fab portion of the antibodies. The Fc portion of IgG antibodies binds certain complement proteins.

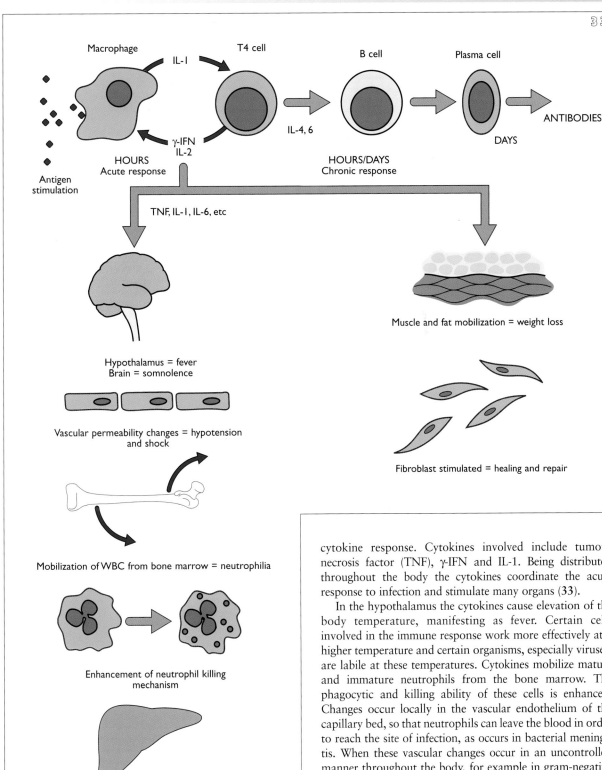

Macrophage   T4 cell   B cell   Plasma cell

IL-1

γ-IFN
IL-2

IL-4, 6

ANTIBODIES

DAYS

Antigen
stimulation

HOURS
Acute response

HOURS/DAYS
Chronic response

TNF, IL-1, IL-6, etc

Muscle and fat mobilization = weight loss

Hypothalamus = fever
Brain = somnolence

Vascular permeability changes = hypotension
and shock

Fibroblast stimulated = healing and repair

Mobilization of WBC from bone marrow = neutrophilia

Enhancement of neutrophil killing
mechanism

Release of acute phase proteins from liver

33 The reaction between the macrophage and T cell initiates the cytokine response. This stimulates the acute response of many organ systems. Chronic stimulation of the cytokine response also has an effect on the body. (γ-IFN: gamma interferon; IL: interleukin; TNF: tumour necrosis factor.)

cytokine response. Cytokines involved include tumour necrosis factor (TNF), γ-IFN and IL-1. Being distributed throughout the body the cytokines coordinate the acute response to infection and stimulate many organs (**33**).

In the hypothalamus the cytokines cause elevation of the body temperature, manifesting as fever. Certain cells involved in the immune response work more effectively at a higher temperature and certain organisms, especially viruses, are labile at these temperatures. Cytokines mobilize mature and immature neutrophils from the bone marrow. The phagocytic and killing ability of these cells is enhanced. Changes occur locally in the vascular endothelium of the capillary bed, so that neutrophils can leave the blood in order to reach the site of infection, as occurs in bacterial meningitis. When these vascular changes occur in an uncontrolled manner throughout the body, for example in gram-negative sepsis, hypotension and septic shock arise. The acute phase proteins, discussed below, are released from the liver.

The effects of prolonged cytokine stimulation, which occurs in chronic infections such as tuberculosis (TB) or 'subacute' endocarditis, is characterized by weight loss, representing the outcome of the cytokine stimulated catabolic process. A low serum albumin is another marker of this catabolism.

Markers of the cytokine response

The acutely ill septic patient can have a high temperature (e.g. 40°C), low blood pressure (e.g. 60/40 mmHg) and laboratory blood tests showing a raised white cell count (WCC), with a neutrophilia in the WCC differential. The clinical parameters and laboratory tests are used to monitor the response of a patient to medical intervention and are an essential adjunct to management of these patients on intensive care units (ICU). The longer the acutely unwell patient has a high fever and low blood pressure (septic shock), in the setting of maximum cardiac and ventilatory support, the less likely the outcome will be favourable.

Markers such as temperature, C-reactive protein (CRP) and erythrocyte sedimentation rate (ESR) are useful in monitoring the effect of treating chronic infections such as subacute endocarditis. The raised ESR is due to the fact that fibrinogen is released from the liver as an acute phase protein. Fibrinogen causes red blood cells (RBCs) to stick to each other, with a faster sedimentation rate. Resolution of a fever after several days of appropriate antibiotics followed by the progressive return of the CRP and ESR to normality are reassuring, and means that the antibiotic regime instituted is likely to be effective in eliminating the infection from the infected heart valve. Some of the parameters commonly used in the management of the infected patient are shown in **34**.

Acute phase proteins

The liver produces the acute phase proteins, which are released under the influence of cytokines and IL-6 in particular. Important acute phase proteins are CRP, mannose binding lectin (MBL) and endotoxin binding protein. Mannose is a constituent of the cell wall of gram-positive and gram-negative bacteria. MBL binds to the mannose residues and as phagocytic cells have receptors for this bound MBL, the bacteria are more readily taken up; this is termed opsonization (**35**).

34		Normal	Acute infection	Chronic infection
Temperature		37°C	40°C	37.8°C
Blood pressure		120/80 mmHg	60/40 mmHg	120/80 mmHg
WCC		$4-10 \times 10^3/\mu L$	$26.4 \times 10^3/\mu L$	$12.4 \times 10^3/\mu L$
Differential count (% neutrophils)		70	95	70
CRP		<10 mg/L	160 mg/L	160 mg/L
ESR		<20 mm/hour	120 mm/hour	120 mm/hour
Albumin		34–48 g/L	25 g/L	20 g/L

34 Some of the clinical and laboratory markers of the inflammatory response, with normal values and examples of those found in acute and chronic infection.
(CRP: C-reactive protein; ESR: erythrocyte sedimentation rate; WCC: white cell count.)

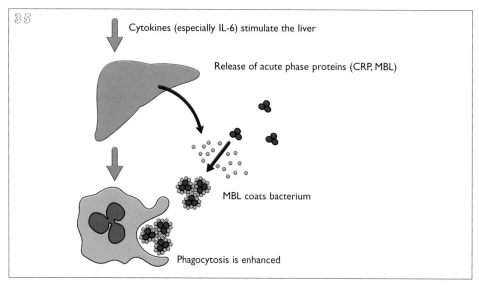

35

Cytokines (especially IL-6) stimulate the liver

Release of acute phase proteins (CRP, MBL)

MBL coats bacterium

Phagocytosis is enhanced

35 Cytokines such as IL-6 stimulate the liver to release the acute phase proteins. Here mannose binding lectin coats the surface of the bacteria, which are then more easily phagocytosed.

Complement

Complement is a group of proteins produced by the liver and cells such as monocytes and macrophages. When IgG antibodies bind to an antigen such as that on the surface of a virus-infected cell, the classic complement cascade is activated. In a specific sequence, complement proteins are cleaved and components of proteins 5–9 form a 'membrane attack complex' that inserts into the cytoplasmic membrane of the infected cell (**36**). The channels produced by these complexes puncture the cell, which dies, thus aborting the replication of the virus in that cell.

In the acute stages of infection before any antibodies are present, the alternate complement pathway can also be activated. Here bacterial cell wall structures can bind component C3 which is cleaved to C3b and C3a, and subsequently C5 is cleaved into C5b and C5a. Bound C3b acts as an opsonin, as phagocytic cells have receptors for C3b (**37**). The C5a produced acts as a chemoattractant, recruiting neutrophils to the site of infection (**38**).

36 When antibodies bind to a cell membrane protein, the classic complement cascade is initiated. The resulting channel allows contents to leak out and the cell dies.

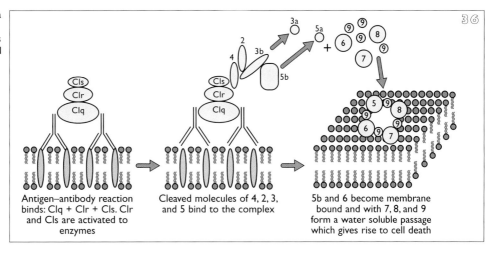

37 Bacterial cell wall components can stimulate the complement cascade via the alternate pathway. C3 is split into C3a and C3b, the latter protein then cleaves C5. Bound C3b is an opsonin and enhances the phagocytosis of bacteria.

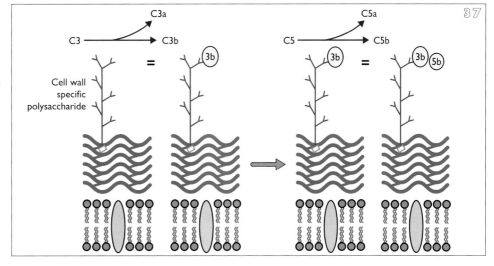

38 Complement component C5a is a powerful chemoattractant and attracts neutrophils and macrophages to the site of infection.

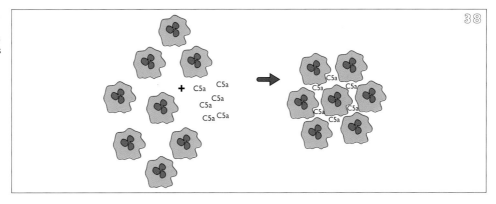

Lipopolysaccharide of the outer membrane of gram-negative bacteria can also activate the alternate pathway; the 'membrane attack complex' that is formed results in the release of endotoxin.

Opsonins such as MBL, C3b and specific antibodies enhance phagocytosis, as phagocytes have receptors for these components when they are bound to bacteria (**39**). Cytokine stimulation of macrophages by the Th-1 cell enhances the expression of the cell surface receptors for C3b and the Fc portion of IgG, increasing the phagocytic properties of cells such as macrophages.

Pathogenic properties of bacteria

Perhaps the most remarkable feature of bacteria is the diversity of their pathogenic characteristics. Even individual bacteria such as *Staphylococcus aureus* have a vast array of weaponry, which includes cell wall proteins, extracellular enzymes and toxins. Some of the pathogenic features of bacteria are shown in **40**, and are discussed in more detail below.

Structural features

A number of important bacteria have an extracellular capsule, which is central to their ability to survive within the host. Capsules have antiphagocytic properties (**41**). If thousands of unencapsulated pneumococci are injected into the peritoneum of a mouse they will have no effect, as the bacteria are rapidly phagocytosed and killed. On the other hand, a few encapsulated bacteria injected into the same site will be able to resist phagocytosis, reproduce and overwhelm the defences and kill the host.

Staphylococcus aureus is able to resist phagocytosis by a specific protein termed protein A. This protein, anchored in the cell membrane, extends through the cell wall to the outside of the cell. The terminal part of the protein is able to bind the Fc portion of IgG antibodies. By coating itself with antibodies in this manner, the organism is protected from the phagocytic actions of the host (**42**).

It is recognized that many bacteria grow in multi-organism biofilms adherent to an inert or living surface. The coagulase-negative staphylococci of the skin form biofilms in

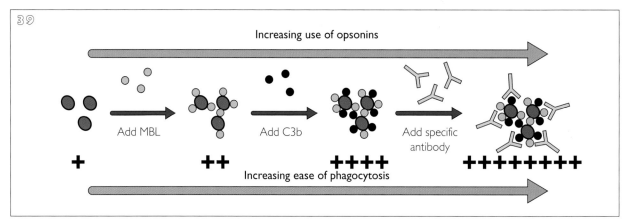

39 Phagocytic cells have surface receptors for mannose binding lectin, C3b, and the Fc portion of IgG antibodies bound to an antigen. The binding of the opsonin to these receptors enhances phagocytosis. (MBL: mannose binding lectin.)

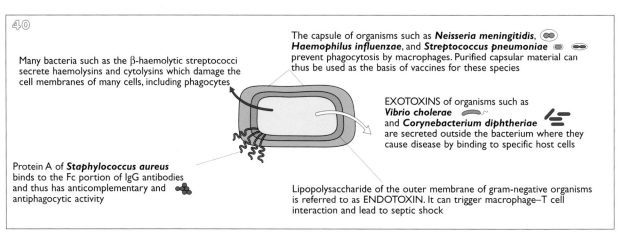

40 This diagram summarizes some important pathogenic properties of bacteria.

long-term central venous catheters, multiplying in the extracellular slime produced by the organism, from where they can seed the blood (**43**). It is often difficult to eradicate these bacteria, as penetration of antibiotics into the slime is poor. The patient with persistent fever, positive central line, and peripheral blood cultures, despite being given appropriate antibiotics, needs to have the central line removed.

Adhesion

An important step for many bacteria in establishing a nidus of infection is the ability to adhere to a surface. In UTI, organisms such as *Escherichia coli* bind to specific receptors on the bladder epithelial cell by adhesins (**44a, b**). Adherent bacteria in the bladder have an advantage over non-adherent bacteria.

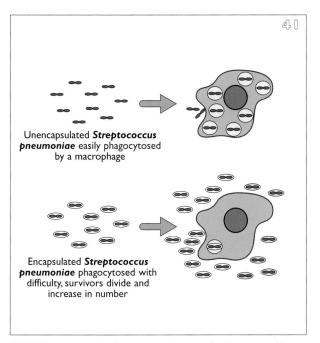

41 While unencapsulated pneumococci are easily phagocytosed by a macrophage, encapsulated organisms can resist phagocytosis and are able to multiply; they may then overwhelm the local defences.

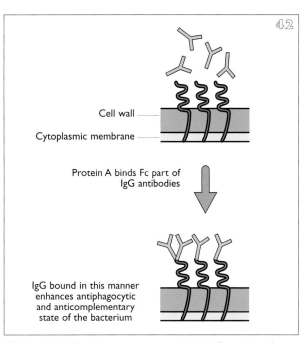

42 Protein A of *Staphylococcus aureus* can bind the Fc portion of IgG antibodies.

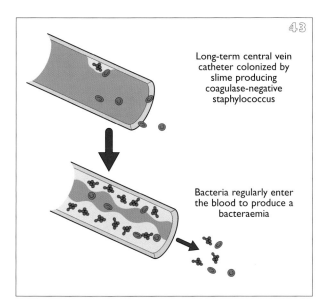

43 Organisms such as the coagulase-negative staphylococci can colonize foreign bodies such as central venous catheters. They exist here surrounded by an extracellular glycocalyx as a biofilm.

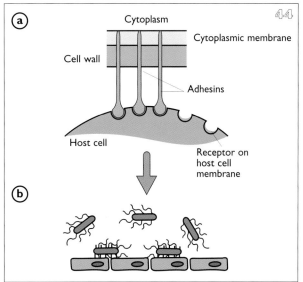

44 (**a**) Many bacteria adhere to the surface of cells by specific adhesins. (**b**) Adherent bacteria have an advantage over non-adherent bacteria in a place such as the bladder, as they are not washed out at micturition.

Secreted proteins

The secretion of extracellular proteins is a significant pathogenic feature of bacteria. *Staphylococcus aureus* secretes the enzyme hyaluronidase. A scratch of the skin may allow resident organisms to enter into the superficial layer of the skin. Hyaluronidase breaks down the hyaluronic acid matrix between the cells, allowing the bacteria to penetrate into deeper layers of the skin (**45**).

Many bacteria such as the β-haemolytic streptococci produce extracellular proteins termed haemolysins. These proteins are able to disrupt host cell membranes by enzymatic or detergent action, resulting in cell death by lysis (**46**). This haemolytic activity is demonstrated in the laboratory by the lysis (clearing) around colonies of bacteria when they are grown on blood agar. Important to the organism is the ability of the haemolysin to disrupt the cytoplasmic membrane of phagocytes, thus compromising the action of these cells. *Listeria monocytogenes* is a small gram-positive bacillus that can cause invasive disease. This organism produces a haemolysin, which degrades the membrane of the phagosome. When phagocytosed, *Listeria monocytogenes* is able to escape into the cytoplasm where it cannot be destroyed (**47**).

Many bacteria secrete proteinaceous exotoxins, which usually consist of an A and B component. The A component is the active part of the toxin, while the B component is responsible for the binding of the toxin to specific receptors on the cell's surface (**48**). *Vibrio cholerae* is an important cause of diarrhoea in underdeveloped parts of the world. The organism is spread via the faecal-oral route through contaminated water. The exotoxin produced by *Vibrio cholerae* binds via component B to receptors on the surface of enterocytes of the bowel. Internalization of the A component results in increased cyclic adenosine monophosphate (cAMP) levels in the cell, which gives rise to water and salt loss; a profuse watery and life-threatening diarrhoea results. Botulism is another exotoxin-mediated disease. *Clostridium botulinum* produces spores, which can survive cooking. If contaminated food is stored for a long period, spores germinate and the vegetative bacteria secrete the neurotoxin responsible for the clinical manifestation of botulism.

Endotoxin

Bacteria such as *Escherichia coli* and *Neiserria meningitidis* can initiate endotoxic shock. Within the outer membrane of gram-negative bacteria is the lipopolysaccharide endotoxin, which can activate the alternate complement pathway (**49a**). The resulting 'membrane attack complex' releases endotoxin, which is bound by endotoxin binding protein, an acute phase protein released from the liver. This complex is then taken up by macrophages. When large numbers of macrophages are activated in this manner, uncontrolled release of cytokines gives rise to endotoxic or septic shock (**49b**).

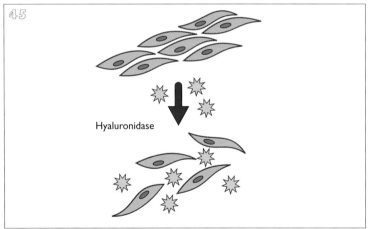

45 In connective tissue, the production of hyaluronidase by *Staphylococcus aureus* allows the organism to spread through the tissue.

Hyaluronidase

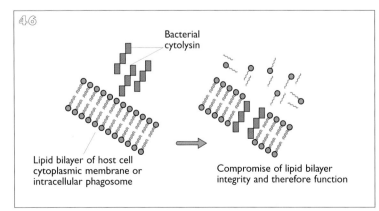

46 Bacterial cytolysins such as the ß-haemolysin of the streptococci can degrade host cell membranes by acting as enzymes or detergents.

Bacterial cytolysin

Lipid bilayer of host cell cytoplasmic membrane or intracellular phagosome

Compromise of lipid bilayer integrity and therefore function

47 *Listeria monocytogenes* produces a cytolysin that enables the organism to escape from the phagosome into the cytoplasm of the macrophage.

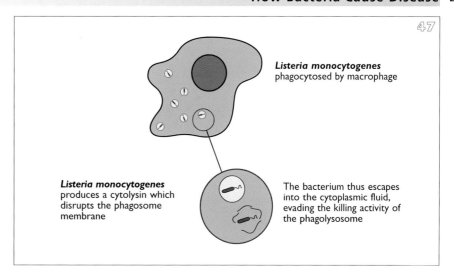

Listeria monocytogenes phagocytosed by macrophage

Listeria monocytogenes produces a cytolysin which disrupts the phagosome membrane

The bacterium thus escapes into the cytoplasmic fluid, evading the killing activity of the phagolysosome

48 The toxin produced by *Vibrio cholerae* binds to specific receptors on the surface of the enterocyte by its B component. The internalized A component increases adenyl cyclase activity. (cAMP: cyclic adenosine monophosphate.)

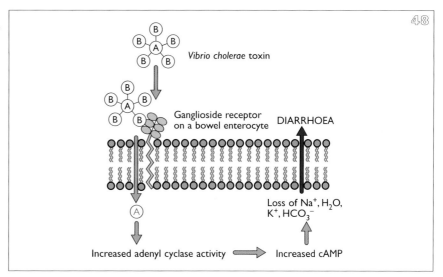

Vibrio cholerae toxin

Ganglioside receptor on a bowel enterocyte

DIARRHOEA

Loss of Na^+, H_2O, K^+, HCO_3^-

Increased adenyl cyclase activity ⟹ Increased cAMP

49 (**a**) Damage to the outer membrane of gram-negative bacteria results in release of lipopolysaccharide (endotoxin). (**b**) Endotoxin/endotoxin binding protein complex (E) binds to macrophages, producing an uncontrolled cytokine response with endotoxic or septic shock.

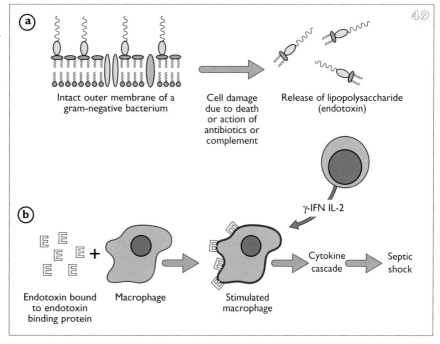

(**a**) Intact outer membrane of a gram-negative bacterium

Cell damage due to death or action of antibiotics or complement

Release of lipopolysaccharide (endotoxin)

γ-IFN IL-2

(**b**) Endotoxin bound to endotoxin binding protein

Macrophage

Stimulated macrophage

Cytokine cascade

Septic shock

Superantigens

Under normal circumstances when an APC and T cell interact, relatively few cells are involved. Toxic shock syndrome (TSS) is caused by toxins such as the pyrogenic toxin of group A streptococcus and the enterotoxins of *Staphylococcus aureus*. These proteins act as superantigens, which cause macrophages and T cells to interact in a non-specific manner (**50**). This results in massive cytokine release, which gives rise to TSS, with fever, hypotension and multi-organ failure.

Immune-mediated diseases

Rheumatic heart disease is relatively uncommon in developed parts of the world but is still important in underdeveloped part of the world. The responsible organism is group A streptococcus, *Streptococcus pyogenes*. Recurrent untreated pharyngitis results in activation of an immune response.

The antibodies produced to the cell wall M protein of the streptococcus cross-react with antigenic determinants on the vascular endothelium of the host. The heart valves are the most important anatomical sites affected, as the high flow rate and turbulence around the valves means the complement deposition and the resulting inflammatory response is likely to cause structural damage to the valve. The healing process results in a thickened and abnormal valve (**51**). Any subsequent damage to the endothelium by turbulence will result in the deposition of platelets and fibrin. Oral streptococci such as *Streptococcus salivarius* entering the blood, following for example manipulation of the teeth by dentistry, can settle in these deposits and initiate the process of infective endocarditis.

Comment

Both immunology and bacterial pathogenesis are broad and detailed subjects, and our understanding of these subjects has progressed dramatically with the advances in modern molecular biology. The outlines presented here are both brief and general. There are many excellent textbooks covering these subjects, which can be browsed in the medical school library or bought in the bookshop.

The *New England Journal of Medicine* has produced a number of excellent reviews on immunology in 2000 and 2001. These are listed below:

Delves PJ, Roitt IM (2000). The immune system. *New England Journal of Medicine* **343**: 37–49.

Delves PJ, Roitt IM (2000). The immune system. *New England Journal of Medicine* **343**: 108–17.

Klein J, Sato A (2000). The HLA system. *New England Journal of Medicine* **343**: 702–9.

Klein J, Sato A (2000). The HLA system. *New England Journal of Medicine* **343**: 782–6.

Mackay I, Rosen FS (2000). Innate immunity. *New England Journal of Medicine* **343**: 338–44.

Von Andrian UH, Mackay CR (2000). T-cell function and migration. *New England Journal of Medicine* **343**:1020–33.

Walport MJ (2001). Advances in immunology: complement. *New England Journal of Medicine* **344**: 1058–66.

Walport MJ (2001). Advances in immunology: complement. *New England Journal of Medicine* **344**: 1140–4.

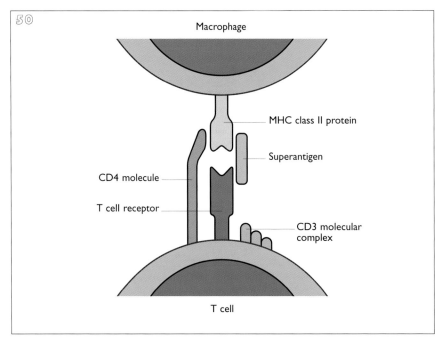

50 Superantigens such as pyrogenic toxin bypass the standard antigen presentation mechanism and uncontrolled cytokine release results in TSS. (TSS: toxic shock syndrome.)

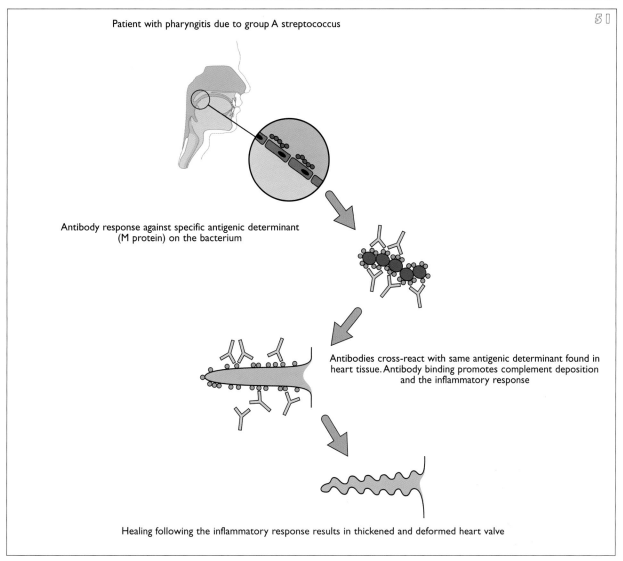

51

Patient with pharyngitis due to group A streptococcus

Antibody response against specific antigenic determinant (M protein) on the bacterium

Antibodies cross-react with same antigenic determinant found in heart tissue. Antibody binding promotes complement deposition and the inflammatory response

Healing following the inflammatory response results in thickened and deformed heart valve

51 Antibodies to the M protein of group A streptococcus cross-react with antigenic determinants of the host. By binding to the endothelium of the heart valves these antibodies initiate an inflammatory response. The resulting healing with fibrosis leads to abnormal valves.

3 Characterization of Bacteria from Clinical Specimens

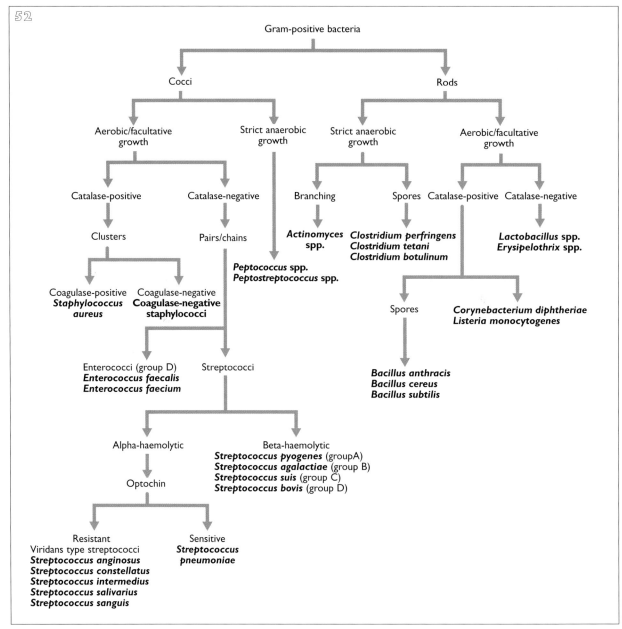

52 Flow diagram showing the classification of gram-positive bacteria.

Introduction

An outline of the classification of gram-positive and gram-negative bacteria is shown in **52** and **53**. Note that this classification uses the gram stain and a number of other simple laboratory tests. One role of the medical microbiology laboratory is to process specimens obtained from patients with suspected infection, in order to isolate and identify relevant bacteria; the information obtained is used to confirm the clinical diagnosis. By determining the antibiotic susceptibility profile of bacteria isolated, the appropriateness of antibiotics being prescribed can be assessed.

It is important that specimens taken are appropriate. Collecting numerous sets of blood cultures from the patient with suspected endocarditis who has already been started on antibiotics is often pointless. A thorough clinical assessment needs to be made and the correct investigations used. Specimens taken carelessly add unnecessary work. Blood cultures contaminated at collection with bacteria derived from the skin can account for as many as 50% of all positive blood cultures processed.

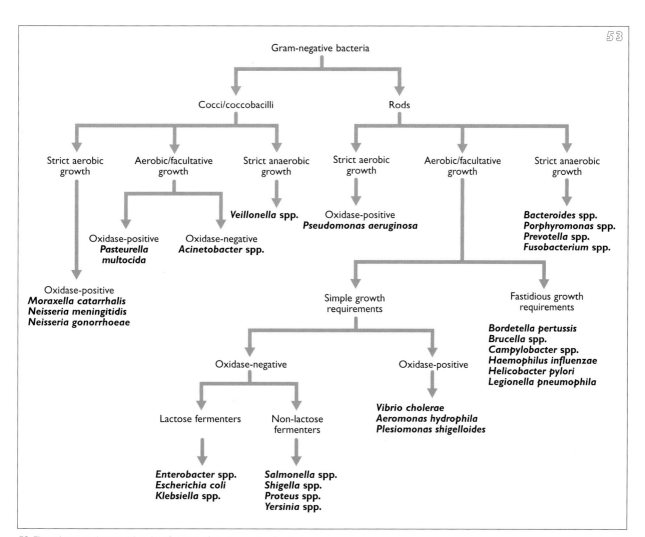

53 Flow diagram showing the classification of gram-negative bacteria.

Some points to bear in mind when collecting specimens for bacteriological processing are shown in **54**. Some of the swabs that can be used for collecting specimens from the genitalia are shown in **55**. Vaginal discharges can be collected using a charcoal transport swab. This needs to be sent to the laboratory promptly in order that the specimen can be examined for labile organisms such as trichomonas. In order to screen for chlamydia, the larger diameter swab is used to obtain an endocervical specimen from female patients. The narrow diameter swab is used for the male patient, and should be inserted 2.0–2.5 cm into the urethra. Both swabs break about 4 cm from the end, enabling the swab to be broken off into the chlamydia transport medium after collection. Herpetic ulcers on the vulva can be carefully opened and sampled with a dry swab, which is then snapped off into viral transport medium. It is also important to use the correct blood bottles for various tests. Red and yellow top tubes, for clotted blood, are used for serology and antibiotic assays, while purple top tubes containing the anticoagulant EDTA are used for the meningococcal PCR test (**56**).

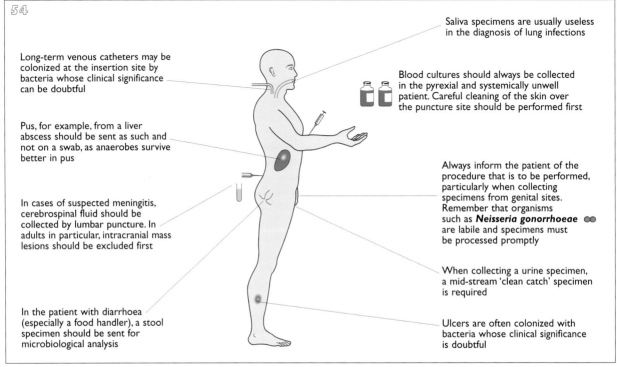

54

Saliva specimens are usually useless in the diagnosis of lung infections

Long-term venous catheters may be colonized at the insertion site by bacteria whose clinical significance can be doubtful

Blood cultures should always be collected in the pyrexial and systemically unwell patient. Careful cleaning of the skin over the puncture site should be performed first

Pus, for example, from a liver abscess should be sent as such and not on a swab, as anaerobes survive better in pus

Always inform the patient of the procedure that is to be performed, particularly when collecting specimens from genital sites. Remember that organisms such as ***Neisseria gonorrhoeae*** are labile and specimens must be processed promptly

In cases of suspected meningitis, cerebrospinal fluid should be collected by lumbar puncture. In adults in particular, intracranial mass lesions should be excluded first

When collecting a urine specimen, a mid-stream 'clean catch' specimen is required

In the patient with diarrhoea (especially a food handler), a stool specimen should be sent for microbiological analysis

Ulcers are often colonized with bacteria whose clinical significance is doubtful

54 Specimen collection from a 'patient', for demonstration purposes only.

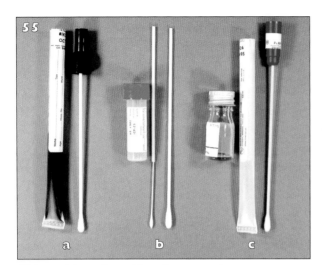

55 Some of the swabs used for collecting genital specimens: (**a**) vaginal discharge, (**b**) chlamydia specimens, and (**c**) those for viral culture.

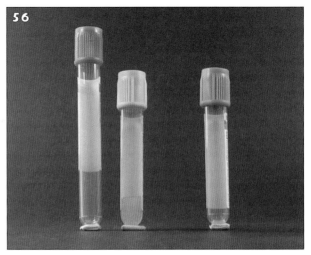

56 Red and yellow topped tubes are used where serum is needed for tests in serology. Purple topped EDTA tubes are used for collecting blood for the meningococcal PCR.

Processing of a specimen

To illustrate how a specimen is processed in the bacteriology laboratory, the example of a specimen of pus aspirated from a liver abscess is used. The most likely bacteria present would be members of the 'normal' bowel flora comprising enterococci, streptococci, 'coliforms', and anaerobes. The first tests performed on the specimen are a gram stain and WCC differential stain (57). A specimen of pus will usually show a large number of neutrophils, and may also reveal a number of gram staining types of bacteria. Gram-positive cocci in chains may be enterococci,

facultative streptococci, or anaerobic streptococci. The gram-negative rods may be 'coliforms' or *Bacteroides* spp.

The specimen is then plated out onto a range of solid (agar) media in order to optimize the growth of all the bacteria. The media used are shown in 58. A portion of the specimen is also inoculated into an 'enrichment' broth of liquid media such as Brain Heart Infusion (BHI) broth, enabling small numbers of bacteria to reproduce. The organisms that grow in the broth will not be numerically representative of those in the original specimen of pus, but enrichment acts as a back-up, especially if antibiotics have

57 The bacteria that may be seen in a gram stain of pus from a pyogenic liver abscess. In the laboratory, media are inoculated that will grow all these bacteria.

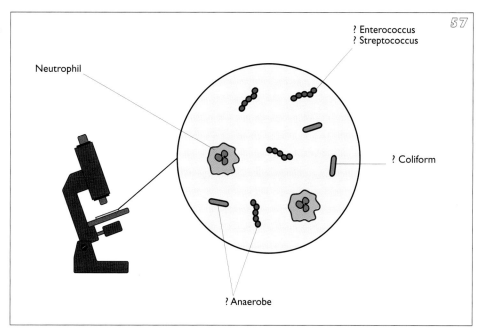

58 A range of solid and liquid media that are commonly used in the bacteriology laboratory.

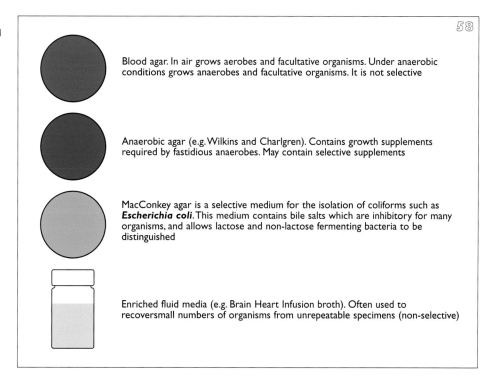

Blood agar. In air grows aerobes and facultative organisms. Under anaerobic conditions grows anaerobes and facultative organisms. It is not selective

Anaerobic agar (e.g. Wilkins and Charlgren). Contains growth supplements required by fastidious anaerobes. May contain selective supplements

MacConkey agar is a selective medium for the isolation of coliforms such as *Escherichia coli*. This medium contains bile salts which are inhibitory for many organisms, and allows lactose and non-lactose fermenting bacteria to be distinguished

Enriched fluid media (e.g. Brain Heart Infusion broth). Often used to recover small numbers of organisms from unrepeatable specimens (non-selective)

damaged the bacteria. When the broth is turbid, indicating growth of bacteria, it is subcultured onto solid media. In the setting of all 'unrepeatable' specimens such as liver abscess pus and tissue biopsies, an enrichment broth should be used. Note that laboratories use a fairly narrow range of culture media to grow most bacteria, as shown in 59. Incubation is usually at 37°C.

When solid culture media are inoculated, a wire loop is used to produce several 'streak' zones (60a). This process dilutes out the organisms in the specimen so that bacteria are sufficiently separated; following multiplication, individual colonies are visible after 18–24 hours of incubation (60b). Each colony represents the reproductive product of one organism and is in essence a 'pure' clone,

59	Bacteria	Atmosphere	Culture medium
	Enterococci	O_2/ANO_2	Blood agar/MacConkey agar
	Beta-haemolytic streptococci	O_2/ANO_2	Blood agar
	Alpha-haemolytic streptococci	O_2/ANO_2	Blood agar
	Streptococcus pneumoniae	O_2/ANO_2	Blood agar
	Staphylococci (all types)	O_2/ANO_2	Blood agar, MacConkey agar
	Haemophilus influenzae	$O_2 + CO_2$	Chocolate agar
	Neisseria meningitidis	$O_2 + CO_2$	Blood agar, chocolate agar
	Neisseria gonorrhoeae	$O_2 + CO_2$	Chocolate agar or enriched blood agar
	Coliforms (Escherichia coli, Klebsiella spp.)	O_2/ANO_2	Blood agar, MacConkey agar
	Salmonella and Shigella spp.	O_2/ANO_2	Blood agar, MacConkey agar, DCA, and XLD agar (selective media)
	Pseudomonas spp.	O_2	Blood agar, MacConkey agar
	Legionella pneumophila	$O_2 + CO_2$	Legionella selective agar
	Bacteroides spp.	ANO_2	Blood agar, anaerobic agar
	Clostridium spp.	ANO_2	Blood agar, anaerobic agar
	Peptostreptococcus spp.	ANO_2	Blood agar, anaerobic agar

59 Most of the organisms considered in clinical practice can be grown on blood or chocolate agar. MacConkey is an example of a selective medium. Special media are needed for an organism such as legionella. (O_2: aerobic [air]; ANO_2: anaerobic; CO_2: 5% CO_2 present).

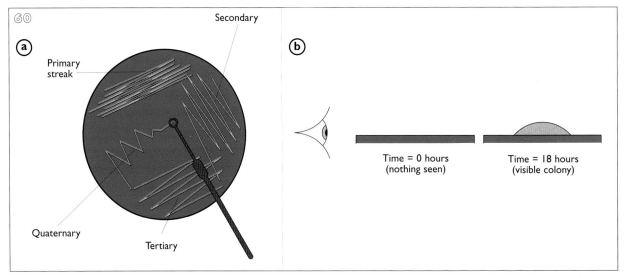

60 (**a**) A 'loop-full' of specimen is inoculated onto agar medium. Usually four 'streaks' are done. (**b**) A progeny of a single bacterium will be visible as a single colony after overnight incubation at 37°C.

which can be used for identification and for antibiotic susceptibility testing. Using such parameters as colonial morphology and atmospheric growth conditions, the biomedical scientist (BMS) will be able to make an initial assessment of the type(s) of bacteria present and will make a decision as to how far different organisms will be processed. Up to three different types of bacteria would warrant each isolate being identified and their antibiotic susceptibility profile determined. However, four or more different bacterial types from the liver abscess pus would usually be reported here as 'faecal flora', and no further work done. Two different coliforms growing on CLED agar, with each having a distinct colonial morphology are shown in **61**.

It is important to remember that a portion of any tissue biopsy should be sent to the histopathology department. In addition, always ask the question 'does this patient have TB?' If this is a possibility, the specimen should be cultured for mycobacteria.

Identification of gram-positive bacteria

Once bacteria have grown up on the solid culture media, a series of simple tests can be used to identify the organism in isolated colonies and a gram stain may be the first test done. Commonly used tests for initial classification of gram-positive bacteria are outlined below. Where necessary, organisms may be fully identified to species level by a range of biochemical tests. Such tests are similar to those discussed with gram-negative coliforms later in this chapter.

Differentiation of streptococci and staphylococci

The catalase test is used to differentiate streptococci (catalase-negative) from staphylococci (catalase-positive). When exposed to hydrogen peroxide, catalase-positive bacteria convert the peroxide to water and gaseous oxygen. There are various ways of determining catalase activity. In the example shown in **62**, a capillary tube containing hydrogen peroxide solution is carefully dipped into a single colony, and if catalase is present, oxygen gas is released and the bubbles observed.

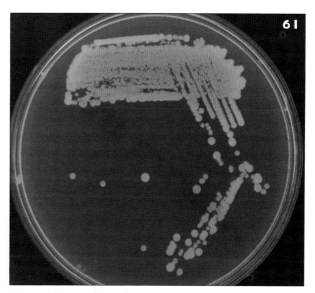

61 Two different coliforms have different colony morphologies as shown here with CLED agar.

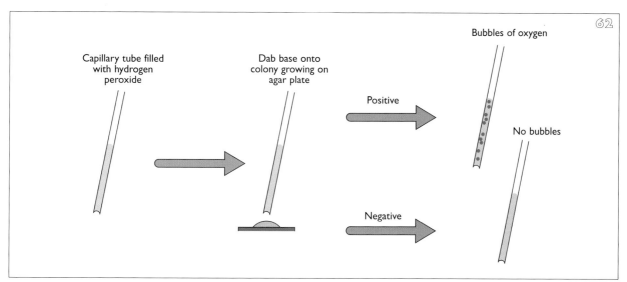

62 An outline of the catalase test.

Differentiation of staphylococci
Coagulase test

The test that is usually done on staphylococcal isolates is the coagulase test. Coagulase is an enzyme that is able to clot plasma in a fashion similar to the thrombin-catalyzed conversion of fibrinogen to fibrin. The test is important in differentiating *Staphylococcus aureus* from the coagulase-negative staphylococci such as *Staphylococcus epidermidis*, which are common skin commensals. The presence of a coagulase-negative staphylococcus in a blood culture would often be considered a skin contaminant, whereas *Staphylococcus aureus* should prompt a reassessment of the patient to determine the possible source.

There are two types of coagulase enzyme, cell bound and free, which are detected by the 'slide' and 'tube' test respectively (**63a, b**). Many commercial kits are available to do tests such as the coagulase. The Oxoid Staphytect™ test uses blue coloured latex beads coated with protein A, fibrinogen, and antibodies to the cell wall polysaccharide of *Staphylococcus aureus*. Coagulase-negative staphylococci will not react with these beads, whereas *Staphylococcus aureus* cross-links the beads by the interaction of the coagulase with fibrinogen, cell wall components with the antibodies, and the fact that protein A binds the Fc portion of the antibodies. Clumping of the beads indicates a positive result (**64**).

DNase test

The identification of *Staphylococcus aureus* can be confirmed by the deoxyribose nuclease (DNase) test, as this organism is DNase-positive and the coagulase-negative staphylococci are DNase-negative. The test relies on the fact

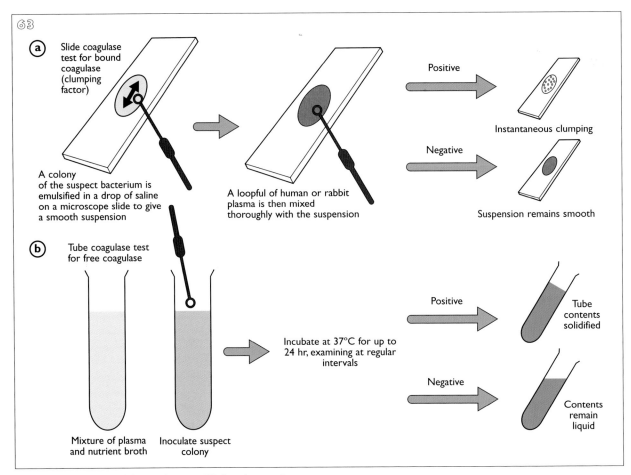

63 An outline of (**a**) the slide coagulase test; (**b**) the tube coagulase test.

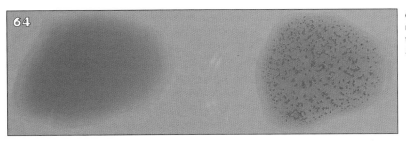

64 A 'loop-full' of two staphylococcal isolates is mixed with Staphytect™ latex beads. Clumping of the blue latex beads identifies one isolate as *Staphylococcus aureus*.

that unhydrolysed native DNA is insoluble and precipitates in strong acid. Agar containing DNA is 'stabbed' with staphylococci and incubated overnight at 37°C. If bacteria in the developing colony secrete the enzyme, DNA will be degraded into soluble nucleotides. After incubation, the plate is flooded with hydrochloric acid. A clear area around a colony, indicating hydrolysis of the DNA, identifies the organism as *Staphylococcus aureus* (**65, 66**).

Identification of streptococci
α- and β-haemolysis
The first step in the classification of streptococci is their haemolytic nature as exhibited on blood agar. Many bacteria produce haemolysins, which are extra-cellular proteins secreted by the cells that degrade lipid membranes. The membrane of red blood cells is also degraded and the lysis of these cells can be seen on blood agar plates. There are two types of haemolysis recognized, α and β. α-haemolysis produces a green discolouration of the agar as a result of incomplete haemolysis of blood cells. β-haemolysis produces a clear zone of haemolysed cells around the bacterial colony.

Optochin test
α-haemolytic streptococci are further subdivided on the basis of the optochin test. *Streptococcus pneumoniae* is sensitive to optochin, while the remainder of the α-haemolytic streptococci are resistant to this compound. This test is shown in **67** and is another example of a simple method to classify an organism to species level.

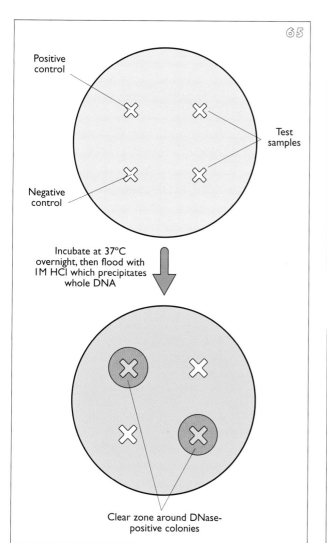

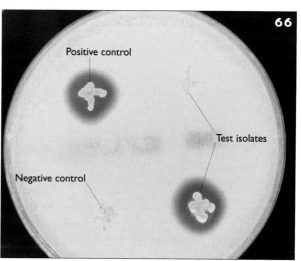

66 A DNase nuclease plate showing both positive and negative results.

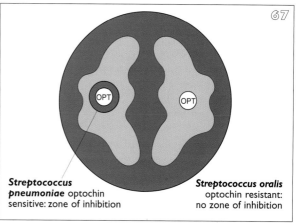

Streptococcus pneumoniae optochin sensitive: zone of inhibition

Streptococcus oralis optochin resistant: no zone of inhibition

65 The deoxyribose nuclease (DNase) test. Staphylococci are inoculated into agar containing macromolecular DNA. Following incubation, addition of hydrochloric acid (HCl) precipitates macromolecular DNA. Around colonies producing DNase, there is no intact DNA and a clear area is seen (**66**).

67 The optochin test to differentiate the α-streptococci. After overnight incubation, a zone of inhibition around the optochin disc identifies the organism as *Streptococcus pneumoniae*.

Lancefield grouping of the β-haemolytic streptococci

The β-haemolytic streptococci are further subdivided on the basis of their cell wall polysaccharide. This 'Lancefield grouping' relies on the extraction of the polysaccharide by enzyme or acid. The procedure used is outlined in **68**. The soluble extract is mixed with latex beads coated with group-specific antibodies; an agglutination reaction identifies the group to which a particular isolate belongs. There are six major groups of β-haemolytic streptococci, termed A, B, C, D, F and G, and within these there are a number of important pathogens, including group A streptococcus, *Streptococcus pyogenes* and group B streptococcus, *Streptococcus agalactiae*.

Examples of α- and β-haemolysis are shown in **69**. Note that when suspected pneumococcus is inoculated onto blood agar, an optochin and an oxacillin disc are placed on the plate. A zone of inhibition to optochin identifies the isolate as pneumococcus. Oxacillin gives an accurate zone size for penicillin, and is used to determine the susceptibility of pneumococcus to penicillin.

Identification of gram-negative bacteria

The gram stain outline of these bacteria, as a rod, coccus, coccobacillus or diplococcus, is useful in making a presumptive identification. The finding of gram-negative diplococci in a CSF specimen collected from a person with meningitis is essentially diagnostic of meningococcal meningitis. Vibrio is a curved organism, while campylobacter and helicobacter are 'seagull' shaped.

Once the bacteria have produced colonies on solid media, the BMS will be able to differentiate 'coliforms', pseudomonas, haemophilus, and other bacterial types. As with gram-positive bacteria, gram-negative organisms can also be classified using simple tests.

Oxidase test

Gram-negative bacteria can be divided into oxidase-positive and oxidase-negative. Oxidase-positive bacteria have cytochrome c (part of the electron transport chain, situated in the cytoplasmic membrane), which is able to convert the colourless agent tetramethyl phenylenediamine to a blue compound. This is an important test as it differentiates oxidase-positive bacteria such as *Pseudomonas aeruginosa*, *Neisseria meningitidis*, and *Neisseria gonorrhoeae*, from the large group of oxidase-negative 'coliforms'. The outline of the procedure is shown in **70** and a positive result in **71**.

X and V test

This simple test is used in most laboratories to differentiate *Haemophilus influenzae* from other haemophilus species. *Haemophilus influenzae* only grows well on the routine diagnostic medium of 'chocolate' agar. Chocolate agar is blood agar where the medium has been heated to 80°C before the plates are poured. This process releases haemin from the lysed red cells into the medium. Haemin (factor X) and NAD (factor V; found in the serum) are essential for the growth of *Haemophilus influenzae*. The test relies on placing paper discs containing either X or V factor and a disc containing both factors on a basic medium such as

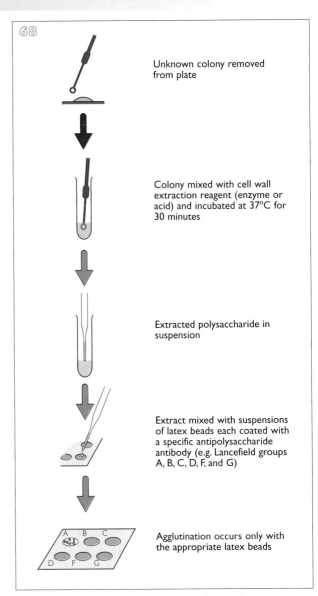

68

Unknown colony removed from plate

Colony mixed with cell wall extraction reagent (enzyme or acid) and incubated at 37°C for 30 minutes

Extracted polysaccharide in suspension

Extract mixed with suspensions of latex beads each coated with a specific antipolysaccharide antibody (e.g. Lancefield groups A, B, C, D, F, and G)

Agglutination occurs only with the appropriate latex beads

68 Lancefield streptococcal grouping of the β-haemolytic streptococci. A positive antibody–antigen reaction is shown by clumps and identifies the group; in this example, group A streptococcus or *Streptococcus pyogenes*.

nutrient agar. *Haemophilus influenzae* will only grow around the XV disc as it has a requirement for both factors. *Haemophilus parainfluenzae* grows around both the XV and V disc, as it only requires the V factor for growth (**72**). Identification of *Haemophilus influenzae* by the X and V test is shown in **73**.

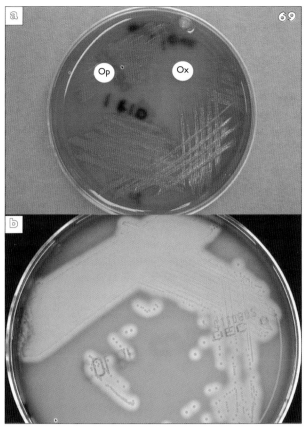

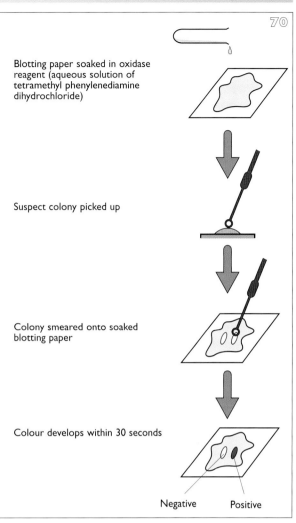

Blotting paper soaked in oxidase reagent (aqueous solution of tetramethyl phenylenediamine dihydrochloride)

Suspect colony picked up

Colony smeared onto soaked blotting paper

Colour develops within 30 seconds

Negative   Positive

69 Blood agar plates showing (**a**) α- and (**b**) β-haemolysis. The α-haemolytic organism is sensitive to optochin (Op) and to oxacillin (Ox), identifying the isolate as a penicillin sensitive pneumococcus.

70 The oxidase test is used to identify gram-negative bacteria. Cytochrome c is able to convert the colourless oxidase reagent to a blue colour, identifying the organism as oxidase-positive.

71 A purple discolouration on oxidase paper indicates an oxidase-positive gram-negative isolate.

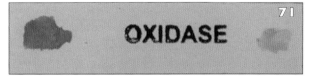

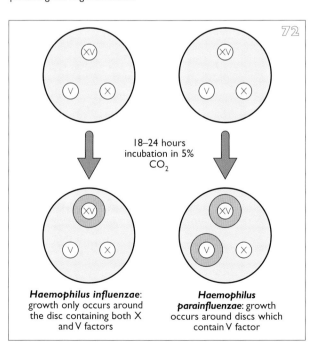

18–24 hours incubation in 5% CO_2

Haemophilus influenzae: growth only occurs around the disc containing both X and V factors

Haemophilus parainfluenzae: growth occurs around discs which contain V factor

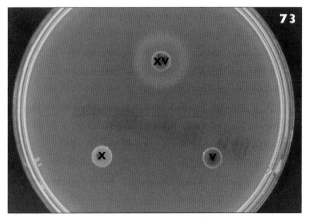

73 An X and V plate identifies *Haemophilus influenzae*.

72 The X and V (NAD) test. *Haemophilus influenzae* is identified by growth around the disc that contains both X and V.

Enterobacteriaceae

The Enterobacteriaceae ('coliforms') are a large family of organisms that contain well recognized pathogens such as *Salmonella* spp. and *Shigella* spp. In addition, organisms such as *Escherichia coli*, which are members of the 'normal' bowel flora, are important causative agents of UTI. This bacterium can be an opportunistic pathogen in the setting of abdominal pathology such as appendicitis, cholangitis, or diverticulitis. *Escherichia coli* O157 is a particular strain that produces an exotoxin, and is the causative agent of haemorrhagic colitis and the haemolytic uraemic syndrome.

A number of simple tests can be used to identify these organisms. Members of the family are classified as either lactose fermenters or non-fermenters. This division relies on the fact that organisms such as *Escherichia coli* produce strong acids from the fermentation of sugars. Acids change the pH indicator in an agar medium such as MacConkey agar to dark red; the bacterial colonies and the agar are thus changed to this colour. On the other hand, non-lactose fermenters such as *Shigella* spp. do not produce strong acids and the colour does not change. A flow diagram of tests used to classify members of this family is shown in **74**.

Biochemical tests

The full identification of 'coliforms' often relies on a series of biochemical tests. As bacteria are able to metabolize (or ferment) certain sugars to acids, growth (turbidity) or a colour change in the medium from alkaline to acid can be used to determine which sugars a particular organism utilizes. The expression of an enzyme such as urease and the detection of end products of metabolism such as indole, a product of tryptophan metabolism, are other tests used. Nowadays a full range of these tests is available commercially, for example the API system produced by BioMerieux. The wells of the 'API strips' are inoculated with a preparation of bacteria from pure culture, incubated overnight, and the biochemical tests either read directly or completed by the addition of various agents. The number code that is produced gives the identification of the organism as outlined in **75**. Three API strips are shown in **76**: (**a**) after inoculation, (**b**) after overnight incubation, and (**c**) after addition of test reagents. The organism here is *Escherichia coli*, which ferments all but two of the sugars, and amongst other test results is indole-positive.

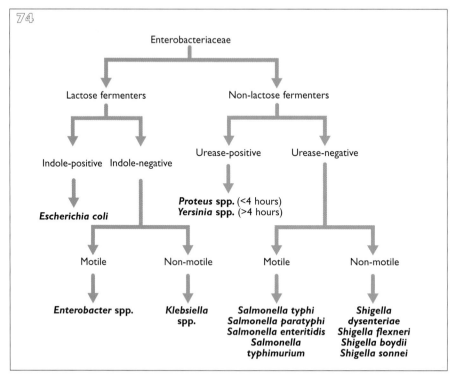

74 Flow diagram of the classification of members of the Enterobacteriaceae. Simple laboratory tests identify most bacteria to genus level.

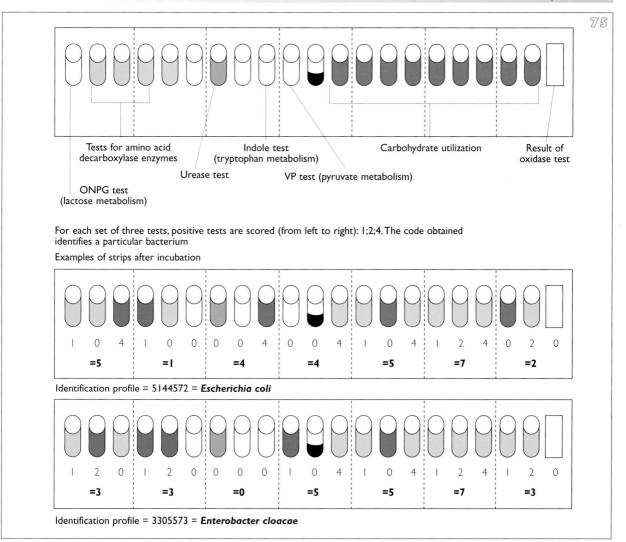

Tests for amino acid decarboxylase enzymes

Indole test (tryptophan metabolism)

Carbohydrate utilization

Result of oxidase test

Urease test

VP test (pyruvate metabolism)

ONPG test (lactose metabolism)

For each set of three tests, positive tests are scored (from left to right): 1;2;4. The code obtained identifies a particular bacterium

Examples of strips after incubation

| 1 | 0 | 4 | 1 | 0 | 0 | 0 | 0 | 4 | 0 | 0 | 4 | 1 | 0 | 4 | 1 | 2 | 4 | 0 | 2 | 0 |
| =5 | | | =1 | | | =4 | | | =4 | | | =5 | | | =7 | | | =2 | | |

Identification profile = 5144572 = *Escherichia coli*

| 1 | 2 | 0 | 1 | 2 | 0 | 0 | 0 | 0 | 1 | 0 | 4 | 1 | 0 | 4 | 1 | 2 | 4 | 1 | 2 | 0 |
| =3 | | | =3 | | | =0 | | | =5 | | | =5 | | | =7 | | | =3 | | |

Identification profile = 3305573 = *Enterobacter cloacae*

75 The API 20E™ (produced by Biomerieux) is an example of a commercially available identification system for bacteria such as coliforms. (ONPG: orthonitrophenyl–β–D–galactopyramoside; VP: Voges–Proskauer.)

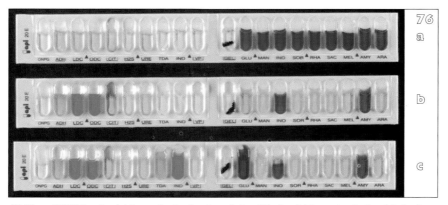

76 Three API 20E strips: (**a**) immediately after inoculation, (**b**) after 24 hours incubation, (**c**) that in (**b**) after the addition of reagents to certain wells. The organism here is *Escherichia coli*. Here the first carbohydrate well (glucose) is also used for the nitrate reduction test.

Serological tests

In addition to biochemical tests, serological tests using specific antibodies are used in the identification of gram-negative bacteria. These tests rely on antibodies raised in animals against pure bacterial isolates. When these antibodies are mixed with a suspension of the bacteria, a clumping or agglutination reaction will occur, and the particular 'serotype' of the organism identified. The various antigens tested for bacteria such as salmonella are shown in **77a**. These are the surface or 'O' antigens and the flagellar or 'H' antigen. The common strain of *Salmonella enteriditis* isolated from stool specimens reacts with antisera O 9 and H gm. This simple test is a quick way of identifying these bacteria (**77b**).

Anaerobic bacteria

Specific diseases caused by anaerobes, such as botulism and tetanus are dealt with in other chapters. For the purpose of this section, it is the anaerobes of the bowel that are considered. As with other bacteria, the gram stain result is part of the initial identification process. Members of the gram-positive clostridia produce heat-stable spores. The position of these spores within the cell is also useful in identification.

By their very nature, anaerobes do not survive in the presence of oxygen, as they are unable to 'detoxify' O_2^- radicals. It is important when collecting a specimen of pus that a sample of the liquid pus is sent, rather than a swab dipped into that pus; survival of the anaerobes will be better in pus. In most laboratories a metronidazole antibiotic disc is placed at the junction of the primary and second streak of the anaerobic blood agar plate (**78a**). The plate is incubated in an anaerobic cabinet, and examined at 48 hours. A zone of inhibition around the metronidazole disc identifies anaerobes, and a report is issued stating 'anaerobes present; metronidazole sensitive' (**78b**). In most circumstances there is no further work done on the organism. Where further identification is deemed necessary, isolates are identified by banks of biochemical tests, such as those in the API system.

Bacteriophage typing

Bacteriophages are viruses which infect bacteria. Infection kills the bacterial cell, which ruptures to release several hundred or more viral progeny, that then infect other bacteria. On an agar plate inoculated with bacteria and virus, the repeated cycles of reproduction initiated by one virus leads to clearings in the bacterial lawn, which are termed plaques. Phages can be very specific, only infecting one strain or subspecies of a bacterium. A range of different phages can thus be used to differentiate certain bacteria further. Phage typing is used to type *Staphylococcus aureus* (including methicillin resistant, MRSA) and *Salmonella enteriditis*.

Enzyme immunoassay

The enzyme immunoassay (EIA), is one of the tests central to medical virology. It is also used in bacteriology for syphilis and legionella serology. An outline of the EIA for detecting antigen or antibodies is shown in **79a, b**. A specific antigen or antibody attached to wells of plastic plates is used to capture the corresponding antibody or antigen in a specimen, usually serum. After incubation and stringent washing, an indicator antibody is added to which an enzyme such as alkaline phosphatase is attached at the Fc end. Following further incubation and washing, the amount of bound indicator antibody is determined by adding the colourless substrate of the enzyme. If enzyme is present, a

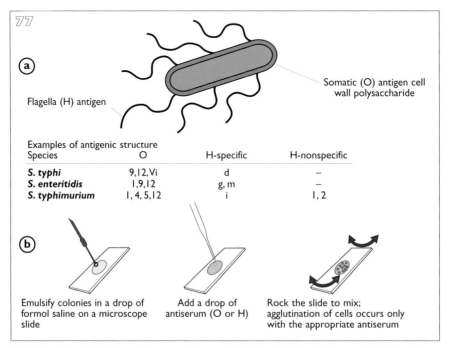

77 (**a**) The O and H antigens that are used for serological identification of salmonella. (**b**) An outline of the slide agglutination test.

78 (a) A metronidazole disc is usually placed on the junction between the primary and secondary 'streak' of the anaerobic blood agar plate.
(b) A zone of inhibition after 48 hours incubation enables 'anaerobes, sensitive to metronidazole' to be reported on the specimen.

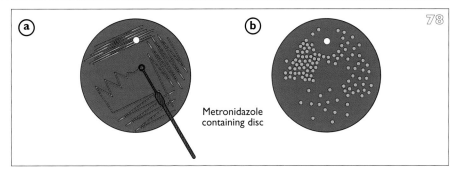

Metronidazole containing disc

79 An outline of the enzyme immunoassay used to **(a)** detect antigen, **(b)** antibody.

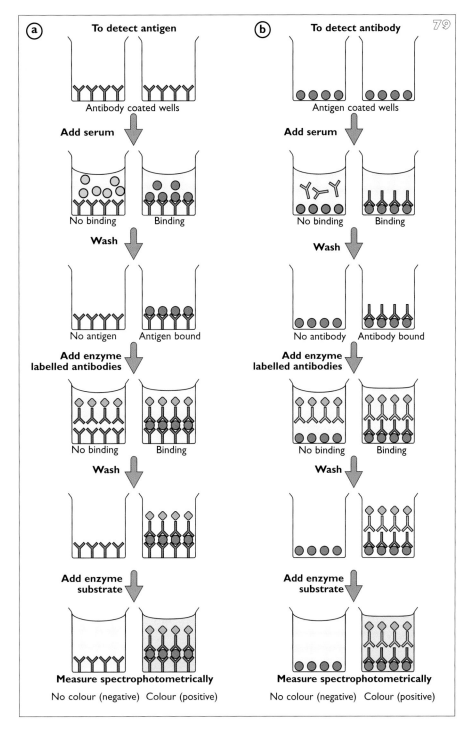

colour reaction is produced proportional to the amount of antibody or antigen in the original specimen. In the case of antibody detection, where a specific human antibody binds to the capture antigen, the presence of this antibody is determined by the addition of, for example, goat anti-human antibodies, to which the enzyme is linked. A 96 well EIA test for chlamydia antigen in genital specimens is shown in **80**. Positive coloured wells are clearly seen.

Complement fixation test

The complement fixation test (CFT) is one of the oldest serological tests and is used to detect antibodies to certain organisms in the serum of a patient. It is still in use today, having an important role in the diagnosis of certain agents responsible for 'atypical pneumonia', including influenza virus, *Chlamydia psittaci*, and *Coxiella burnetii*. There are several steps in the test. Initially, a known antigen is mixed with serum and if this serum contains the specific antibodies they will bind to the antigen. Complement is then added and if an antigen–antibody reaction has taken place, this will also be bound. Sheep RBCs that have been 'sensitized' with specific antibodies to the RBC are subsequently added, and if there is no free complement, the RBCs remain intact and settle out as a pellet in the well; this is a positive result (**81a**). If there was no antigen–antibody reaction in the first step, free complement will attach to the sensitizing antibodies on the RBCs; the complement cascade will then lyse these cells. A diffuse flocculation will be visible in the wells; this is a negative result (**81b**). A photograph of a CFT test plate is shown in **82**.

Polymerase chain reaction

One of the most useful developments in molecular biology in the late 1900s was the PCR, which has revolutionized modern medicine. The method relies on the fact that all organisms have unique sequences that make up their genomes, be they DNA or RNA. If an organism is present in a specimen in very small numbers, the PCR will amplify a specific sequence into a detectable signal. In order to do this, short primer sequences, a heat-stable DNA polymerase, and an excess of nucleotides are needed. By repeated cycles of primer annealing, DNA synthesis and denaturation, an exponential reaction is produced. The end-product, produced within several hours, can be identified by agar gel electrophoresis (**83**). DNA molecules have the same charge to mass ratio, and migrate through an agar gel under the influences of an electric current on the basis of size. By using control DNA molecules and molecular weight markers, a specific amplified DNA sequence can be identified when the gel is stained.

The PCR has many uses in diagnosis. It can be used to amplify and identify TB in CSF obtained from the patient with suspected TB meningitis. A useful PCR is that for meningococcus where the organism can be identified to serogroup level in blood or CSF. PCR is widely used in medical virology for detecting viruses such as cyto-megalovirus (CMV), herpes simplex virus (HSV), hepatitis B virus (HBV) and HIV. Both qualitative and quantitative tests exist. A quantitative HIV PCR is particularly useful for monitoring the viral load in patients infected with HIV who are taking antiviral chemotherapy.

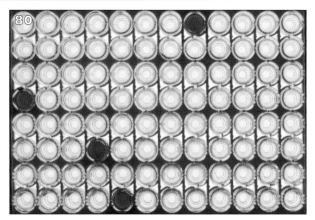

80 A chlamydia enzyme immunoassay, clearly showing the reaction of positive (coloured) samples.

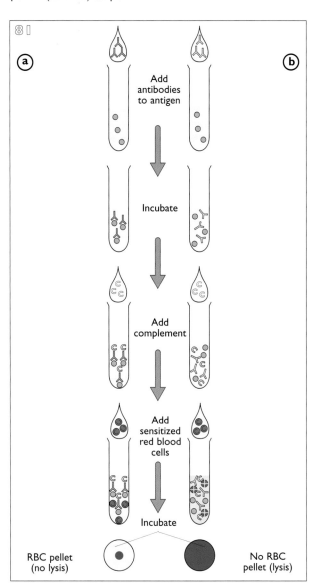

81 The complement fixation test. In (**a**) the antigen and antibody react and complement is bound; the added red blood cells (RBCs) are not lysed and settle out as a pellet. In (**b**) there is no antibody–antigen reaction, complement is not bound and it then binds to the added sensitized antibodies of the RBCs, which lyse.

82 An example of the complement fixation test. A positive result is identified where a pellet of red blood cells (RBCs) is seen. The diffuse settling of lysed RBCs is a negative result.

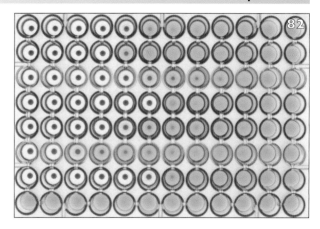

83 The polymerase chain reaction. Repeated cycles of denaturation, primer annealing and deoxyribonucleic acid (DNA) synthesis lead to exponential production of the target DNA that can be identified by gel electrophoresis. Specimen A is positive, specimen B is negative.

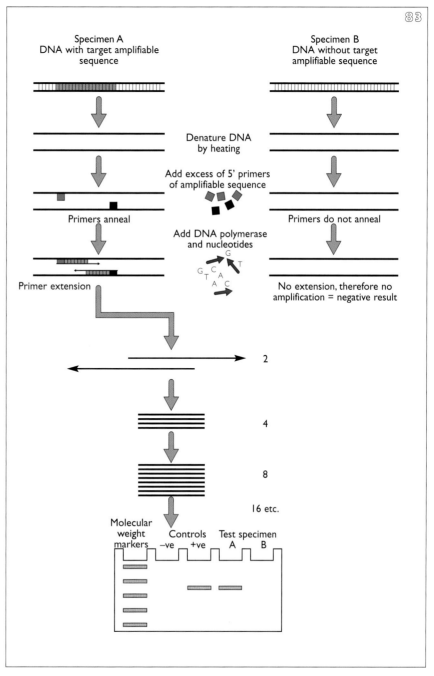

Comment

This chapter has briefly covered the common techniques used to identify bacteria. Serological tests and the new molecular based methods such as PCR are an essential part of the laboratory repertoire. Further information on all these techniques can be found in general microbiology textbooks. For more detailed information, books such as the five comprehensive volumes of Topley and Wilson's *Microbiology and Microbial Infections* can be used; these books are usually found in the medical microbiology departmental library.

It is important to have an appreciation of the work of the medical microbiology laboratory, which processes a wide range of specimens in order to identify bacteria, viruses, fungi, and parasites. The work of a typical laboratory, processing some 200,000 specimens per annum, may break down as follows: urine samples (35%), wound swabs (15%), high vaginal swabs (10%), blood cultures (6%), faeces (3%), sputa (3%), antibiotic assays (3%), virology and serology (15%), and others, including referral of specimens to Reference laboratories (10%). In general it takes 24–48 hours to produce an interim or final result for the majority of specimens. The medical micro-biologist should telephone the initial results on specimens from which 'alert organisms' are isolated. This includes group A streptococci isolated from wounds and tissues and all positive TB microscopy and culture results. Initial microscopy results on all positive blood cultures should also be communicated to a member of the clinical team.

Health care workers should use the laboratory responsibly. Inappropriately collected specimens are a waste of time and resources. For example, a member of the medical staff should take blood cultures and antibiotic assays at the correct time. Leaving the collection of such specimens to the routine morning round of the phlebotomist is not correct procedure. Most hospitals have ward-based computer systems and the health care worker must have responsible access to this. It is important to use this service to review the results of all specimens sent from a patient before contacting the laboratory for further advice and information.

A limited after-hours service is available for the processing of urgent specimens. This should be restricted to the examination of specimens such as pus or CSF, where a positive gram stain result may influence the antibiotics prescribed for the patient. In addition, labile organisms from these sites need to be processed for culture as soon as possible.

4 Use of Antibiotics

Introduction

The clinical assessment of a patient should influence correct antibiotic prescription. It is therefore important to have an appreciation of the bacteria that are likely to be causing a particular infection. For example, one organism such as meningococcus may be considered in a case of bacterial meningitis and a single antibiotic such as cefotaxime prescribed. In peritonitis due to a ruptured colonic diverticulum, all the bacteria of the bowel flora should be considered. Agents effective against gram-positive streptococci, gram-negative 'coliforms', and gram-positive and gram-negative anaerobes would be prescribed. Cefuroxime and metronidazole, or three agents such as ampicillin, gentamicin, and metronidazole,

can be used. Another alternative would be a broad-spectrum agent such as co-amoxiclav, which may be given in combination with gentamicin. Any regime needs to be modified when bacteria are isolated from specimens and when it is clinically appropriate to do so.

In addition to considering the correct antibiotics to prescribe, it is important to appreciate the pharmacokinetics of the agents, their route of excretion, penetration into various body compartments, and toxicity (**84**). Attention should be given to renal and liver function, as antibiotics are excreted or metabolized by these routes. An estimation of renal function should be part of standard patient care, and the urea and electrolyte (U+E) results used to calculate creatinine clearance. RIF, isoniazid (INH), and

84 The 'body' outline shows a number of important principles to bear in mind when prescribing antibiotics. (AAD: antibiotic-associated diarrhoea.)

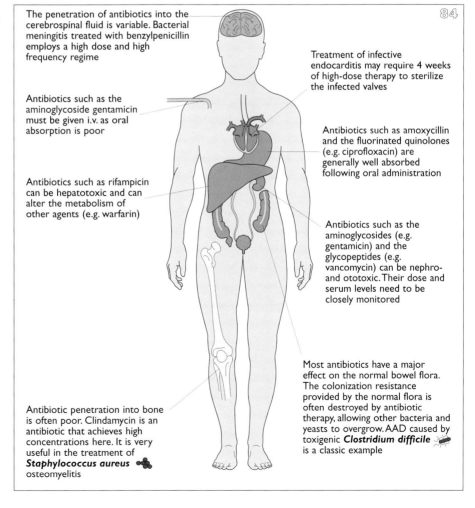

The penetration of antibiotics into the cerebrospinal fluid is variable. Bacterial meningitis treated with benzylpenicillin employs a high dose and high frequency regime

Antibiotics such as the aminoglycoside gentamicin must be given i.v. as oral absorption is poor

Antibiotics such as rifampicin can be hepatotoxic and can alter the metabolism of other agents (e.g. warfarin)

Antibiotic penetration into bone is often poor. Clindamycin is an antibiotic that achieves high concentrations here. It is very useful in the treatment of ***Staphylococcus aureus*** osteomyelitis

Treatment of infective endocarditis may require 4 weeks of high-dose therapy to sterilize the infected valves

Antibiotics such as amoxycillin and the fluorinated quinolones (e.g. ciprofloxacin) are generally well absorbed following oral administration

Antibiotics such as the aminoglycosides (e.g. gentamicin) and the glycopeptides (e.g. vancomycin) can be nephro- and ototoxic. Their dose and serum levels need to be closely monitored

Most antibiotics have a major effect on the normal bowel flora. The colonization resistance provided by the normal flora is often destroyed by antibiotic therapy, allowing other bacteria and yeasts to overgrow. AAD caused by toxigenic ***Clostridium difficile*** is a classic example

pyrazinamide (PZA), which are used in the treatment of TB, can be hepatotoxic. It is prudent to monitor liver function tests (LFTs) in patients taking these agents, and to review treatment promptly when LFTs deteriorate. By inducing liver enzymes, RIF can alter the metabolism of other agents. One example is its effect in compromising the action of the oral contraceptive. Female patients taking RIF and an oral contraceptive must be advised of the likelihood of failure of the latter agent, and the need to use alternative forms of contraception while taking this antibiotic.

The duration of antibiotic therapy depends on the infection. It is appropriate to treat meningococcal sepsis for 5 days with the correct antibiotic. On the other hand, prosthetic heart valve endocarditis caused by a coagulase-negative staphylococcus usually warrants 6 weeks of therapy. Tuberculous meningitis is treated for at least 9 months. What-ever the infection and the duration of treatment, it is essential to bear in mind that most, if not all, antibiotics can have some side-effects. In addition, the unnecessary and prolonged use of antibiotics has been an important contribution to the international problem of antibiotic resistant bacteria. The policy of antibiotic use must be to keep any regimen as narrow spectrum as possible and as short as possible.

Antibiotic susceptibility tests

While antibiotics are often prescribed empirically, one of the main functions of the medical microbiology laboratory is to determine the antibiotic susceptibility of bacteria from clinical isolates. This is for several reasons. First, to ensure that the antibiotics given are appropriate for the organisms isolated and second, to maintain a database for the general antibiotic susceptibility profile in hospitals and the community. Methicillin sensitive (MSSA) and methicillin resistant *Staphylococcus aureus* (MRSA) are examples. On a cardiothoracic unit where the incidence of MRSA is negligible it would be reasonable to treat a suspected staphylococcal bacteraemia with flucloxacillin. If the incidence of MRSA is high, it would be reasonable to prescribe vancomycin initially. The regimen would be continued or modified the next day when the staphylococcus from the blood culture had been fully identified and its antibiotic susceptibility determined.

Minimum inhibitory concentration

The minimum inhibitory concentration (MIC) is the fundamental test in determining the sensitivity of a bacterium to an antibiotic. An outline of the procedure is shown in **85**. A dilute suspension of bacteria is inoculated into tubes, each

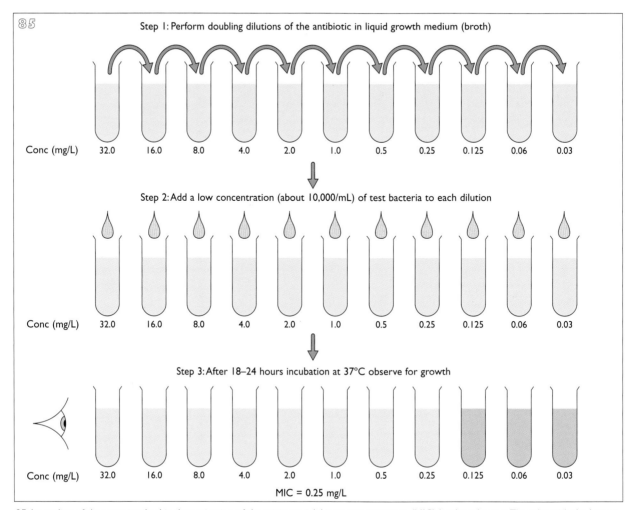

85 Step 1: Perform doubling dilutions of the antibiotic in liquid growth medium (broth)

Conc (mg/L) 32.0 16.0 8.0 4.0 2.0 1.0 0.5 0.25 0.125 0.06 0.03

Step 2: Add a low concentration (about 10,000/mL) of test bacteria to each dilution

Conc (mg/L) 32.0 16.0 8.0 4.0 2.0 1.0 0.5 0.25 0.125 0.06 0.03

Step 3: After 18–24 hours incubation at 37°C observe for growth

Conc (mg/L) 32.0 16.0 8.0 4.0 2.0 1.0 0.5 0.25 0.125 0.06 0.03

MIC = 0.25 mg/L

85 An outline of the steps involved in determination of the minimum inhibitory concentration (MIC) by the tube test. The tube with the lowest concentration of antibiotic that shows no visible growth (turbidity) gives the MIC value.

containing a different concentration of the antibiotic being tested. The highest antibiotic concentration used in the tube test is usually 32 mg/L. The range from 32 mg/L and below is relevant, as it is within this range that antibiotics are usually effective in the blood, fluids and tissues, and where their toxic effects are usually minimal. After overnight incubation, the MIC is determined by examining for growth of bacteria in each tube, indicated by turbidity or 'cloudiness'. The lowest concentration of the antibiotic that inhibits growth is the MIC; in the example in **85**, the MIC is 0.25 mg/L. A photograph of a tube MIC is shown in **86**.

Minimum bactericidal concentration

Another test that can be done is determination of the minimum bactericidal concentration (MBC). Here a loop-full of medium from each of the tubes from the MIC test which shows no turbidity, is inoculated onto agar. Any growth on these agar plates shows that organisms from the

initial inoculum have been inhibited but not killed by the antibiotic; in the example in **87**, the MBC is 1.0 mg/L. If bacteria survive in the tubes that are more than two dilutions above the MIC, e.g. 4.0 mg/L, the bacteria are considered 'tolerant' to the antibiotic. This is an important concept in treating bacterial endocarditis caused by streptococci and enterococci, which can be tolerant to penicillin or amoxycillin alone. In order to be killed, they must be treated with a synergistic combination of agents, for example amoxycillin and gentamicin. The rationale here is that the β-lactam agent damages the cell wall sufficiently to allow gentamicin, at the therapeutic concentration used, to reach and cross the cytoplasm membrane, which it could not do if the organism's cell wall was intact. Note that the streptococci and enterococci are not oxidative organisms and do not have the mechanisms necessary to pump aminoglycosides across the cell membrane, as discussed below in relation to oxidative gram-negative bacteria.

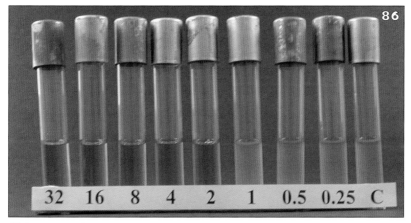

86 Photograph of a tube minimum inhibitory concentration; the result here is 2.0 mg/L. (C: control.)

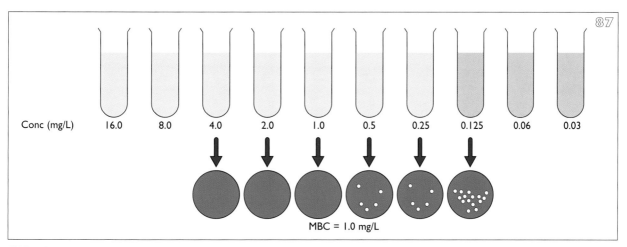

87 For the minimum bactericidal concentration (MBC) a loop-full of broth from each tube showing no turbidity is plated. The lowest concentration of antibiotic where there is no growth of bacteria on the plates determines the MBC.

Disc susceptibility test

The MIC and MBC tests are cumbersome and are not suitable for routine high volume work. Most laboratories use the disc susceptibility test. Here, cellulose discs impregnated with a standard amount of an antibiotic are placed on agar plates inoculated with the organism to be tested. As the bacteria multiply during overnight incubation, the antibiotic diffuses into the agar. A zone of inhibition is produced proportional to the susceptibility of that organism to a particular antibiotic (88, 89). Using standardized criteria, the size of the zone of inhibition equates to the organism's resistance or sensitivity to the antibiotic. Results are usually reported as 'resistant' or 'sensitive'; occasionally the term 'intermediate' may be used. Note that in the example shown in 88, isolate B is resistant to amoxicillin. This is due to production of β-lactamase, which degrades the β-lactam ring of amoxycillin and related antibiotics, including penicillin and ampicillin, rendering them inactive.

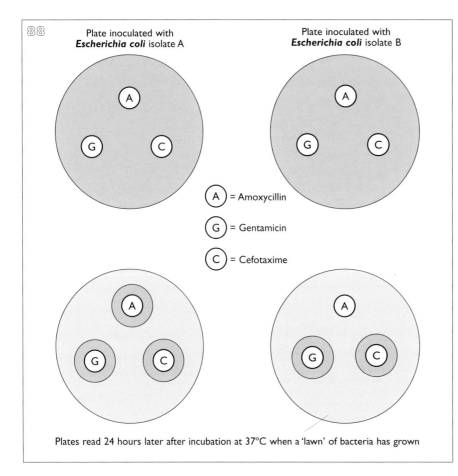

88 Disc susceptibility testing. The example here shows that isolate B is resistant to amoxycillin.

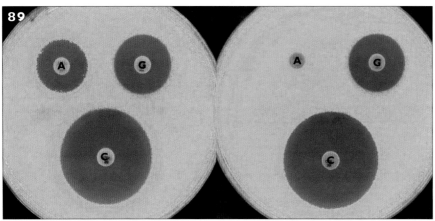

89 Photographs of two isolates of a 'coliform'. Both are sensitive to gentamicin (G) and cefotaxime (C). One is resistant to amoxycillin (A) due to β-lactamase activity.

Etest™

A recent advance in susceptibility testing has been the development of the Etest™. This ingenious test employs a strip of material incorporating an exponential gradient of an antibiotic from one end to the other. The strip is placed on an inoculated plate (**90a**). As the organism multiplies, the antibiotic diffuses out of the strip. The rate of diffusion is proportional to the concentration at a particular point, and this will determine the zone of inhibition. The MIC can be read from the scale, as shown in **90b**. A photograph of an Etest is shown in **91**. While the test is more expensive and labour intensive than the disc method, it is useful for determining the MIC of selected organisms. For example, laboratories may monitor the MIC values of *Streptococcus pneumoniae* isolates in a region where the prevalence of isolates with reduced susceptibility to penicillin is regarded as significant.

Antibiotic kinetics

In order to help the natural defenses of the body control and defeat a bacterial infection, an antibiotic must be present at an effective concentration and for sufficient time. The concentration should usually exceed the MIC by some factor. However, the concentration of the antibiotic must not be so high that it is toxic to the patient. The kinetics of a single dose of an antibiotic is shown in **92**. Most antibiotics have a half-life of 1–2 hours and, following distribution into the various body compartments, are eliminated from the body, usually by the kidneys or liver. As shown in **92**, when the MIC value of an antibiotic for a particular organism is superimposed on the graph, the antibiotic concentration falls below the MIC value after a certain period, and in most circumstances the next dose should be given by that time.

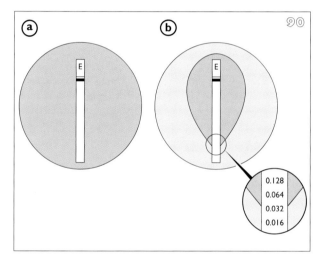

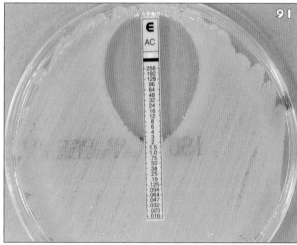

90 The Etest™. (**a**) A strip containing a logarithmic range of concentrations of an antibiotic is placed on an inoculated plate. (**b**) After incubation, the minimum inhibitory concentration is determined by reading the scale; here, 0.032 mg/L.

91 An amoxycillin Etest™ tested against a sensitive 'coliform'.

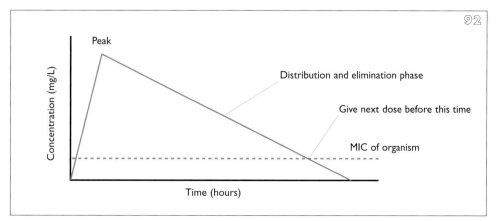

92 The kinetics of a single dose of an antibiotic. Superimposing the minimum inhibitory concentration (MIC) of the antibiotic for a particular organism shows that the timing of doses is important to maintain antibiotic levels that will inhibit or kill bacteria.

Pharmacokinetics of the β-lactams

The β-lactam antibiotics include the penicillins, cephalosporins, and carbapenems. These agents interfere with the cross-linking of the peptidoglycan of the cell wall. Their effectiveness depends on the concentration exceeding the MIC during a course of treatment, and continually saturating the active sites of the PBP (**93a**). If the concentration is below the MIC, the active sites of the PBP are not saturated and bacteria may survive (**93b**). The half-life of the various β-lactams differs considerably, from about 1 hour for benzylpenicillin and 8 hours for ceftriaxone. If either of these two agents is used to treat meningitis caused by a penicillin sensitive isolate of *Streptococcus pneumoniae*, the regime for benzylpenicillin could be 1.2 g 3 hourly, whereas that for ceftriaxone could be 2 g once a day (**94a, b**).

Pharmacokinetics of the aminoglycosides

The mode of action of the aminoglycosides such as gentamicin is different from the β-lactams. The aminoglycosides inhibit protein synthesis and thus need to reach the cytoplasm. Simplifying the overall mechanism, these antibiotics bind to the outer membrane of the cell wall of gram-negative bacteria and then enter aerobically metabolizing organisms such as *Pseudomonas aeruginosa* and coliforms by a specific mechanism. Aerobic metabolism in these bacteria requires a terminal electron transport chain situated in the cytoplasmic membrane. This process results in the extrusion of hydrogen ions, giving rise to an electrochemical gradient across the membrane. This gradient is used as the proton motive force to generate adenosine triphosphate (ATP) (**95a**). The aminoglycosides probably enter the cell by this force and, consequently, gram-negative bacteria in the aerobic form of metabolism have no option but to pump the agent into their cytoplasm. If there is a sufficient concentration of the aminoglycoside outside the cell, the bacteria will in effect commit molecular suicide (**95b**). Under acidic or anaerobic conditions, hydrogen ions outside the cell reduce the ability of the cell to pump out its own hydrogen ions. The electrochemical gradient is diminished and entry of the antibiotic into the cell is progressively reduced. Presumably when facultative 'coliforms' are in an environment where the oxygen supply becomes diminished, they will switch from aerobic respiration to fermentation. In this situation, the activity of an aminoglycoside will be compromised.

In order to gain the best use of the aminoglycosides, the 'once daily' or 'pulse dose' regimen is now in use. This replaces the traditional 'three times a day' regimen. In the 'pulse dose' regimen a dose of 5–7 mg/kg/lean body weight is given over 30 minutes. This gives the reassurance that the patient has sufficient aminoglycoside in the blood for at least 24 hours. The kinetics of the 'pulse dose' and 'three times a day' or 't.d.s' regimens are shown in **96**. This shows that for a period of up to around 1 hour in the pulse dose regimen, the MIC of susceptible gram-negative bacteria is exceeded by a factor of >10, which more or less guarantees effective killing of susceptible bacteria in the blood. The fact that the concentration falls below the MIC before the next dose is given is not usually important, as any surviving bacteria remain crippled until the next dose by a 'post-antibiotic effect'.

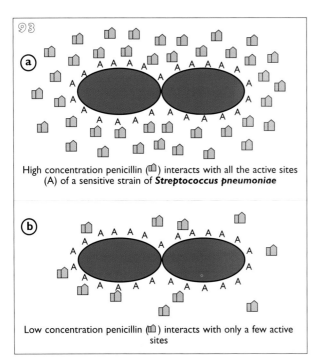

High concentration penicillin (🏠) interacts with all the active sites (A) of a sensitive strain of **Streptococcus pneumoniae**

Low concentration penicillin (🏠) interacts with only a few active sites

93 (a) The effectiveness of the β-lactam antibiotics requires concentrations that saturate all the available active sites (A) of the penicillin binding protein on the cell membrane. **(b)** If concentrations are too low the organisms will be able to survive and multiply.

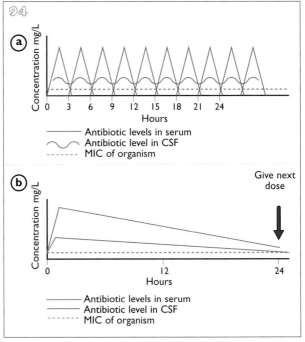

Antibiotic levels in serum
Antibiotic level in CSF
MIC of organism

Give next dose

Antibiotic levels in serum
Antibiotic level in CSF
MIC of organism

94 (a) In order to achieve adequate levels of benzylpenicillin in the cerebrospinal fluid (CSF), frequent doses must be given. **(b)** The half-life of ceftriaxone is 8 hours and a single 2 g dose can be given daily.

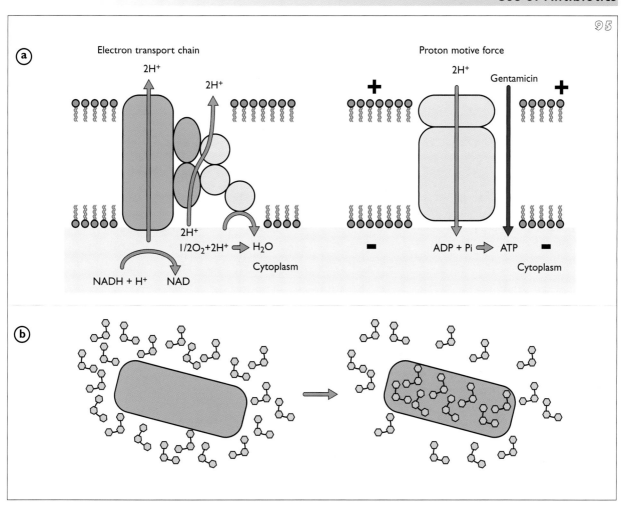

95 (a) When growing aerobically, gram-negative organisms use the terminal electron transport chain. The proton motive force is 'parasitized' by aminoglycosides. **(b)** Susceptible oxidative bacteria are unable to resist the entry of the aminoglycoside into the cell. (ADP: adenosine diphosphate; ATP: adenosine triphosphate; NAD: factor V.)

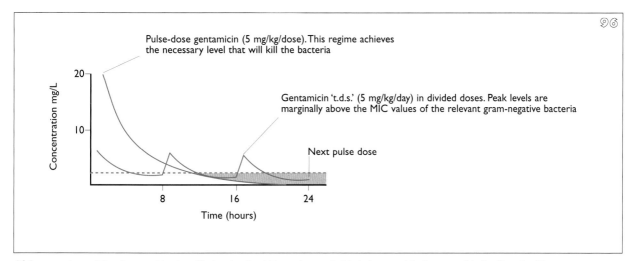

96 A comparison of the pharmacokinetics of 'pulse dose' and 'three times a day' (t.d.s.) gentamicin. A post-antibiotic effect should prevent any survivors recovering once the antibiotic concentration falls below the minimum inhibitory concentration (MIC). (Modified from Nicolau DP *et al.* (1995) Experience with a once-daily aminoglycoside program administered to 2184 adult patients. *Antimicrobial Agents and Chemotherapy* **39**, 650–655.)

Importance of estimating renal function

Use of the 'pulse dose' regimen should prompt the prescribing doctor to determine the patient's renal function, as the aminoglycosides are excreted via the kidneys. The formula below gives a reasonable estimate of creatinine clearance. It takes into account important factors such as sex, age, lean body mass, and current serum creatinine (**97**). The use of such a formula should be routine. After calculating the clearance, the interval between doses is determined:

$$\text{Creatinine clearance} = \frac{170 - \text{age in years} \times \text{wt (kg)}}{\text{serum creatinine}}$$

The value of 170 applies to male patients below 70 years of age. For males above this age and all female patients, use 160 and 150 respectively. (Cronberg S [1994]. Simplified monitoring of aminoglycosides. *Journal of Antimicrobial Chemotherapy* **34**: 819–27.)

If clearance is:
100–60 mL/min the interval between doses is 24 hours.
59–40 mL/min the interval between doses is 36 hours.
39–20 mL/min the interval between doses is 48 hours.

This formula can also be used to determine the dose interval when the glycopeptide vancomycin is used. The usual adult dose is 1 g 12 hourly. If the creatinine clearance is for example 50 mL/min, the interval between doses can be increased to 24 hours.

Antibiotic assays

When a patient is prescribed an aminoglycoside or the glycopeptide vancomycin, the serum concentration of the agent needs to be assayed at regular intervals. This is to ensure that there are effective levels, and that the agent is not accumulating as both can cause renal and oto-toxicity. Using the pulse dose regimen for gentamicin, a pre-dose level can be collected before the second or third dose, and should be less than 1.0 mg/L. In the setting of normal renal function, the first vancomycin pre-dose specimen should be collected before the fourth or fifth dose; the value should be between 5 and 10 mg/L. Any value above these pre-dose values requires a reassessment of the patient's renal function, and if the antibiotic is continued, the interval between doses should be increased. Post-dose levels are not regarded as useful.

Commonly used antibiotics, their range of action and bacterial resistance mechanisms

In this section a number of antibiotics are discussed in relation to their range of activity, and the mechanisms whereby bacteria become resistant to them. The organisms represented in **5** are presented in the relevant diagrams in this chapter on the 'x' axis. The antibiotics are considered here in general terms to have good, average, or poor activity against particular bacteria. Good means that the antibiotic is usually the correct choice; average means that the agent can be used, but there are better alternatives, and poor means that the agent should not be used. Below average means that the antibiotic is really not appropriate for a particular organism.

For simplicity, the organisms used in the diagrams each have a specific antibiotic susceptibility pattern. *Staphylococcus aureus* is the isolate which is resistant to benzylpenicillin, ampicillin, and amoxycillin due to β-lactamase activity, but is flucloxacillin (methicillin) sensitive (MSSA). *Escherichia coli* and *Haemophilus influenzae* are represented by isolates that do not produce β-lactamase, whereas *Klebsiella pneumoniae* is representative of all isolates of this organism which do produce a plasmid-mediated β-lactamase. The other coliforms include isolates of enterobacter and citrobacter which can be found in the hospital environment. These bacteria produce a chromosomal β-lactamase that is not inhibited by β-lactamase inhibitors such as clavulanic acid. Isolates that synthesize large quantities of the enzyme can inactivate essentially all the cephalosporins.

The most widely used class of antibiotics is the β-lactam antibiotics. They act on the active site of the PBP, the enzymes that are responsible for the cross-linking of the peptidoglycan chain of the cell wall.

Benzylpenicillin, ampicillin/amoxycillin, co-amoxiclav, piperacillin/tazobactam, and flucloxacillin

The range of activity of these antibiotics is shown in **98a–e**. There is little difference between ampicillin and amoxycillin, except that the oral bioavailability of amoxycillin is about 95%, double that of ampicillin. Benzylpenicillin, ampicillin, and amoxycillin have their

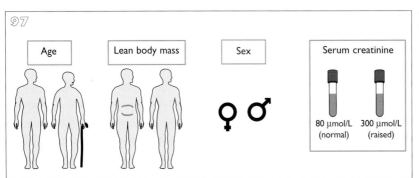

97 Four important parameters to remember when calculating renal function.

Age   Lean body mass   Sex   Serum creatinine

80 µmol/L (normal)   300 µmol/L (raised)

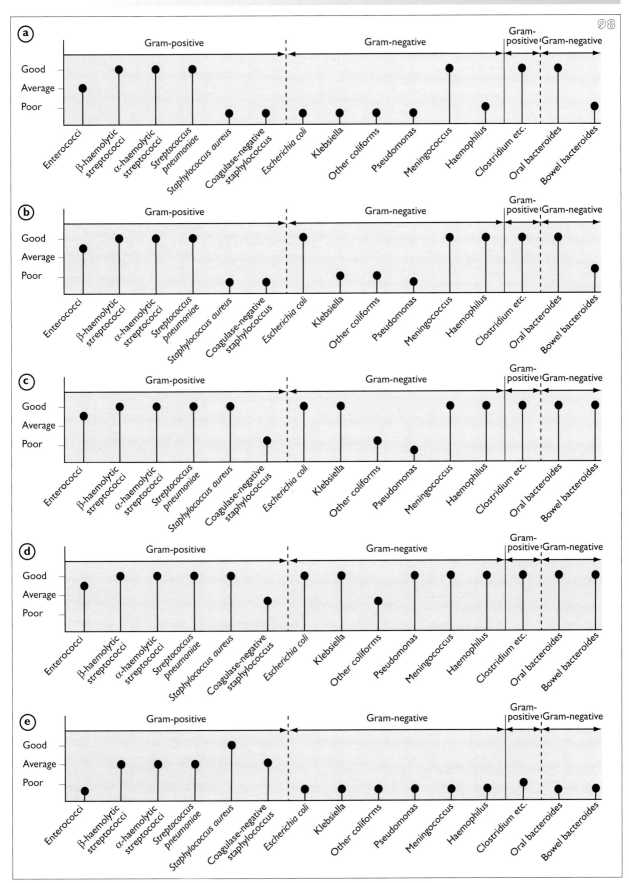

98 The range of activity of (**a**) benzylpenicillin, (**b**) ampicillin/amoxycillin, (**c**) co-amoxiclav, (**d**) piperacillin/tazobactam, (**e**) flucloxacillin.

activity compromised because many bacteria have developed resistance to them by the action of β-lactamase enzymes. These enzymes can be coded by chromosomal or plasmid genes and cleave the C–N bond of the β-lactam ring, rendering the antibiotic useless. In gram-positive bacteria the enzyme is secreted outside the cell, but with gram-negative bacteria the enzyme is largely retained in the periplasmic space. An example of these enzymes is the plasmid coded TEM-1 β-lactamase found in about half of all isolates of *Escherichia coli*.

Co-amoxiclav is a combination of amoxicillin and clavulanic acid. Clavulanic acid is a β-lactam derivative, but has no useful antibiotic activity. It does however, have high affinity for the β-lactamase enzyme produced by *Staphylococcus aureus*, members of the Enterobacteriaecae such as *Escherichia coli* and *Klebsiella* spp., and *Haemophilus influenzae*. Clavulanic acid binds to the active site of the β-lactamase enzyme, neutralizing its enzymatic activity (**99**). The amoxycillin component thus remains in its active form and can bind to the PBP. Enterobacter and citrobacter produce a chromosomally-mediated β-lactamase that is not inactivated by inhibitors such as clavulanic acid.

It is worthwhile to note that β-lactams such as piperacillin have good activity against *Pseudomonas aeruginosa*. Piperacillin combined with the β-lactamase inhibitor tazobactam provides a useful broad-spectrum antibiotic whose activity is similar to co-amoxiclav, but in addition has antipseudomonal activity (**98d**). This agent should usually have restricted use to specialist units such as intensive care. Piperacillin achieves very high concentrations in the unobstructed biliary tract.

Flucloxacillin, active against MSSA, was developed as a commercial modification of benzylpenicillin. The modified R1 side chain sterically prevents the β-lactamase enzyme from cutting the C–N bond of the β-lactam ring (**100a**); the activity of the antibiotic is thus retained (**100b**). Flucloxacillin has reasonable activity against streptococci and can be used to treat mild cases of cellulitis, which may be caused by *Staphylococcus aureus* and streptococci.

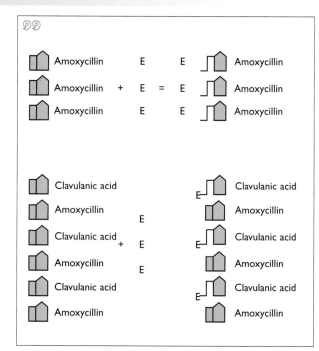

99 The β-lactamase enzyme (E) inactivates amoxycillin. By binding to the active site of the β-lactamase enzyme, clavulanic acid protects the amoxycillin from the action of the ß-lactamase.

Methicillin resistant *Staphylococcus aureus* (MRSA)

MRSA is a major problem in many hospitals. In 2000, a survey in England and Wales showed that over 40% of blood cultures positive with *Staphylococcus aureus* were MRSA, compared to less than 5% in 1992. Similar changes have been noted in other parts of the world. This trend will lead to increasing use of the glycopeptides vancomycin and teicoplanin, resulting in further selection of glycopeptide resistant enterococci and other resistant gram-positive organisms.

Resistance to methicillin in MRSA is due to the production of a different PBP, coded by the chromosomal *mec* gene. This PBP, termed 2a' does not bind β-lactam antibiotics such as methicillin (the agent used in laboratory tests) and flucloxacillin (**101**). The 2a' protein is able to carry out peptidoglycan cross-linking and bacterial growth continues. With resistance common to other agents such as the macrolides and fluorinated quinolones, the range of antibiotics used to treat MRSA infections is reduced, and a glycopeptide is often the antibiotic of choice.

Penicillin resistant pneumococci

Penicillin resistant pneumococci are common in certain parts of the world, and in parts of Europe and Africa they account for over 50% of pneumococcal isolates. Pneumococci are classed as being sensitive (MIC <0.1 mg/L), intermediate (MIC 0.1–1.0 mg/L), or resistant (MIC >1.0 mg/L). Reduced susceptibility to penicillin arises by an unusual mechanism. Pneumococci can take up free DNA from their environment, for example in the upper respiratory tract, a process termed transformation. Only DNA from related oral (viridans) streptococci is used, which is then exchanged by DNA recombination. Antibiotic selection pressure makes it logical for a pneumococcus to take up and exchange DNA from related streptococci, which code for PBP that have reduced susceptibility to penicillin (**102a**). As shown in **102b**, there is a progression in the development of resistance as successive genes coding for different PBP are transformed, giving rise to the selection of resistant organisms.

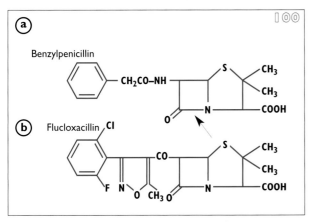

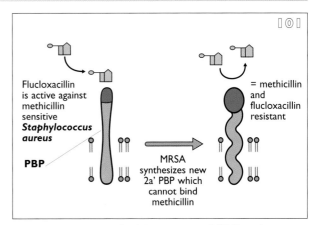

100 (**a**) The arrow shows the site of action of the β-lactamase enzyme. (**b**) In the case of flucloxacillin, modification of the side chain results in a structure that sterically inhibits the enzyme.

101 Methicillin resistant *Staphylococcus aureus* (MRSA) synthesizes a new penicillin binding protein (PBP) 2a'. While the other penicillin binding proteins are inactivated by flucloxacillin, the 2a' protein takes over the cross-linking function.

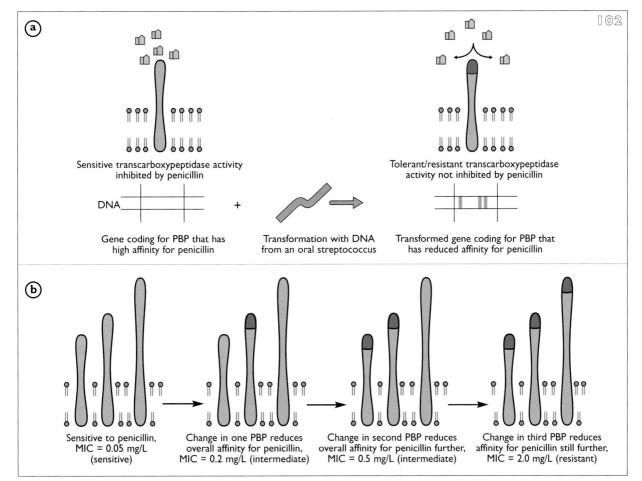

102 Reduced susceptibility to penicillin in pneumococcus is due to production of penicillin binding proteins (PBPs) that have reduced affinity for penicillin. (**a**) The genes coding for the PBP are transformed by deoxyribonucleic acid (DNA) of related streptococci. (**b**) Consecutive transformation steps leads to organisms that have intermediate and then resistant profiles. (MIC: minimum inhibitory concentration.)

Cephalosporins

This class of antibiotics consists of a large number of agents. The range of activity of cefuroxime, cefotaxime, and ceftazidime are shown in **103a–c**. These agents are often used in the hospital setting. Note that none of these antibiotics are effective against the enterococci. Ceftazidime is active against *Pseudomonas aeruginosa*. The cephalosporins are usually resistant to the standard plasmid-mediated β-lactamase produced by 'coliforms' such as *Escherichia coli* and *Klebsiella* spp. However, their high use in a hospital can select out strains of these bacteria, which produce a plasmid-mediated 'extended-spectrum β-lactamase' (ESBL) that can inactivate cephalosporins.

Carbapenems

The carbapenems have no sulphur residue in the five-carbon thiazolidine ring, hence their name. There are several of these broad-spectrum agents in use, including imipenem, meropenem, and ertapenem (**104**). Meropenem has marginally better gram-negative activity than imipenem, while ertapenem has limited activity against pseudomonas. Carbapenems are resistant to the β-lactamase enzymes produced by many bacteria, including ESBL producing 'coliforms'. Previously their use was restricted to the intensive care setting, but the increasing problem of 'ESBL producers' in the hospital and the community has widened their use. Ertapenem is given 'once-daily' and is thus a useful agent to consider in the setting of a 'home care' intravenous antibiotic service in the community. Meropenem can be used for meningitis caused by 'coliforms' and pseudomonas, as therapeutic levels are achieved in the CSF.

Acquired resistance to imipenem in particular can arise in pseudomonas. Passage of the antibiotic across the outer membrane is via a specific hydrated porin channel D2. A single point mutation in the D2 gene produces a protein that prevents entry of the antibiotic, and thus resistant isolates of *Pseudomonas aeruginosa* arise (**105**).

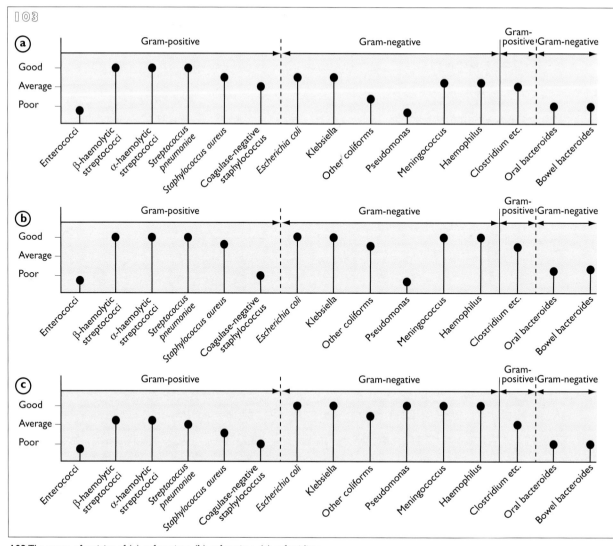

103 The range of activity of (**a**) cefuroxime, (**b**) cefotaxime, (**c**) ceftazidime.

Glycopeptides vancomycin and teicoplanin

Coagulase-negative staphylococcal infections are commonly found in situations where long-term indwelling catheters are used, such as in leukaemic or chronic ambulatory peritoneal dialysis (CAPD) patients. The glycopeptides are frequently used to treat these infections. The range of activity of vancomycin and teicoplanin is shown in **106**; note that these antibiotics are only effective against gram-positive bacteria. The reason for this is that their large molecular size prevents them from crossing the outer membrane of most gram-negative bacteria, and thus they cannot reach the site of action of peptidoglycan synthesis.

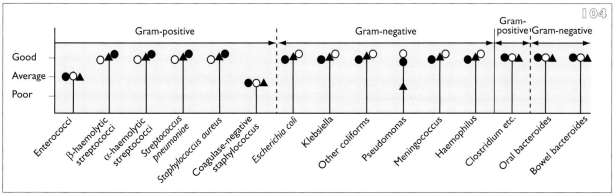

104 The range of activity of ertapenem (▲), imipenem (●), and meropenem (○).

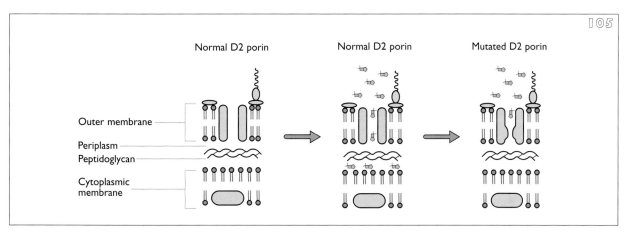

105 Acquired resistance to imipenem in *Pseudomonas aeruginosa*. The antibiotic gains access to the periplasmic space via a D2 porin. Mutation in the gene coding for the porin protein changes the structure of the channel, blocking passage of the antibiotic.

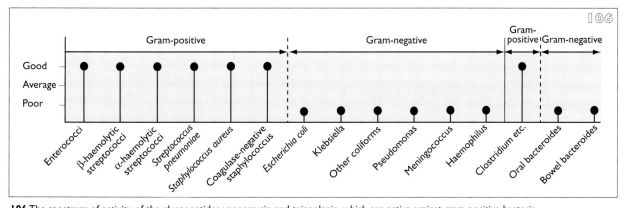

106 The spectrum of activity of the glycopeptides vancomycin and teicoplanin, which are active against gram-positive bacteria.

It was thought that gram-positive organisms would be unable to become resistant to these agents, as their mode of action (preventing the 'building block' of the peptidoglycans from entering the correct site) was considered an essential step that could not be bypassed (**107a**). However, glycopeptide resistant enterococci such as vancomycin resistant enterococcus (VRE) are now well recognized. These organisms are able to add a terminal lactose residue at the end of the peptide side chain, replacing the terminal alanine. This prevents the antibiotic from binding to the 'building block', and peptidoglycan synthesis can continue (**107**). Glycopeptide tolerance/ resistance has been reported in both coagulase-positive and coagulase-negative staphylococci; the implications of this resistance are obvious.

Aminoglycosides

The most commonly used aminoglycoside is gentamicin, although netilmicin, tobramycin, and amikacin are used occasionally. The range of activity of gentamicin is shown in **108**. Note that apart from *Staphylococcus aureus*, the main use of these agents is the treatment of infections involving the 'coliforms' and *Pseudomonas aeruginosa*. The aminoglycosides have no useful activity against anaerobes or facultative bacteria such as coliforms growing anaerobically for the reasons outlined before in this chapter.

Metronidazole

Metronidazole is commonly used to treat anaerobic infections (**109**). Metronidazole probably enters all bacterial cells. True anaerobes have a very negative redox potential value and under these conditions metronidazole is converted into toxic intermediates that bind to and degrade the chromosomal DNA of the organism. As this physiological environment is essential for the existence of anaerobes, these organisms have no option but to commit 'molecular suicide' when exposed to metronidazole.

There are other agents with useful activity against anaerobes, such as co-amoxiclav, piperacillin/tazobactam, and the carbapenems. Their activity resides in neutralizing the action of β-lactamase enzymes. However, all these antibiotics have broad-spectrum activity (**98c, d, 104**). Clindamycin and RIF also have activity against anaerobes (**110, 111**).

The fluorinated quinolones

Fluorinated quinolones such as ciprofloxacin and norfloxacin have useful activity against the gram-negative 'coliforms', pseudomonas, meningococcus, gonococcus, and haemophilus. The range of activity of ciprofloxacin is shown in **112**. The fluorinated quinolones can be alternatives for treating the 'atypical' pneumonia organisms named in the following macrolide section. Agents such as levofloxacin and moxifloxacin also have useful gram-positive activity.

Macrolides

The macrolides include erythromycin, clarithromycin and azithromycin. These agents have useful activity against streptococci and MSSA (**113**). They are thus alternatives to consider in the treatment of infections caused by these organisms in penicillin allergic patients.

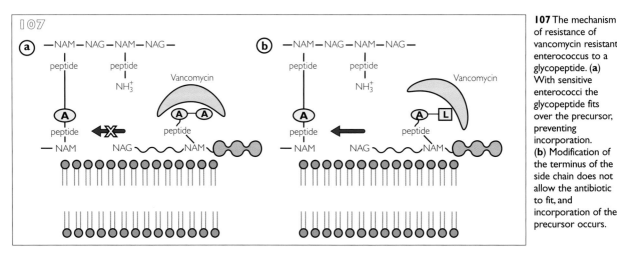

107 The mechanism of resistance of vancomycin resistant enterococcus to a glycopeptide. (**a**) With sensitive enterococci the glycopeptide fits over the precursor, preventing incorporation. (**b**) Modification of the terminus of the side chain does not allow the antibiotic to fit, and incorporation of the precursor occurs.

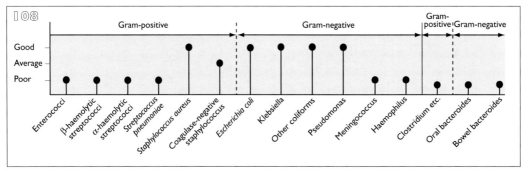

108 The range of activity of gentamicin.

109 The range of activity of metronidazole.

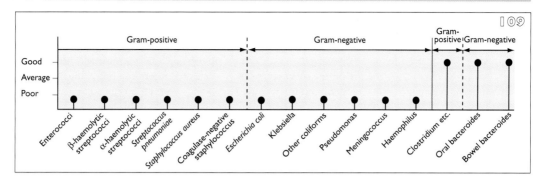

110 The range of activity of clindamycin.

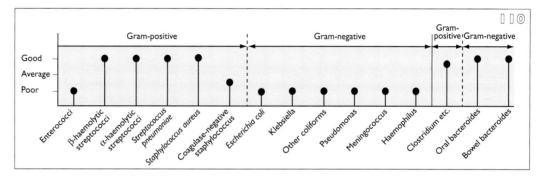

111 The range of activity of rifampicin.

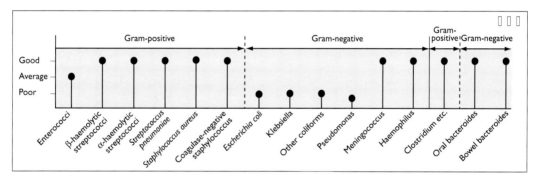

112 The range of activity of ciprofloxacin.

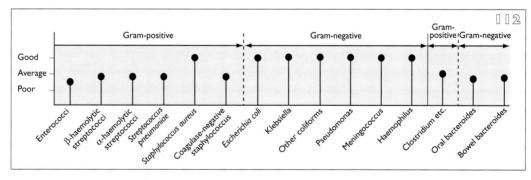

113 The range of activity of the macrolide erythromycin.

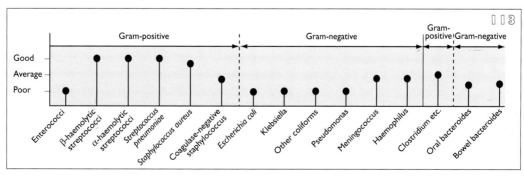

The macrolides also have good activity against the causative agents of 'atypical pneumonia' such as mycoplasma, *Legionella pneumophila*, *Chlamydia pneumoniae*, *Chlamydia psittaci* (psittacosis), and *Coxiella burnetii* (Q fever). It is usual to consider the use of one of these agents when admitting a patient with severe community acquired pneumonia (CAP). Although more expensive than traditional antibiotics, a single dose of azithromycin is useful in the treatment of sexually transmitted disease caused by *Neisseria gonorrhoeae* and *Chlamydia trachomatis*.

Clindamycin

Although in a different class of antibiotics, clindamycin has similar biological properties to the macrolides, and inhibits protein synthesis in susceptible bacteria by the same mechanism. Clindamycin has good oral bioavailability and penetrates well into tissues. It is useful in the treatment of osteomyelitis and brain abscesses, particularly in the patient who has an allergy to penicillin which may rule out the use of β-lactam antibiotics. Clindamycin is considered by some to be an important cause of *Clostridium difficile* antibiotic-associated diarrhoea, and for this reason its general use may be limited. The range of activity of clindamycin is shown in **110**.

Rifampicin

RIF acts by inhibiting the initiation of RNA synthesis. RIF is recognized as one of the most important agents in the treatment of TB, but can be used against a number of other bacteria including gram-positives and anaerobes. The agent is well absorbed and penetrates well into tissues. It can be hepatotoxic, and of particular relevance is its ability to induce liver microsomal enzymes. This can lead to increased turnover of agents such as steroids, including the oral contraceptive, and the anticoagulant warfarin.

RIF should have restricted use and should not be used alone, as bacteria can become resistant to this antibiotic relatively quickly. The range of activity of RIF is shown in **111**.

Chloramphenicol

Chloramphenicol inhibits protein synthesis. This antibiotic is not often used systemically because of its association with the rare condition of aplastic anaemia. However, having good oral bioavailability and tissue penetration it is very useful in circumstances such as a brain abscess. The range of activity of chloramphenicol is shown in **114**.

Tetracyclines

The tetracyclines include tetracycline itself and doxycycline. These agents inhibit protein synthesis. They are important agents in the treatment of genital infections caused by chlamydia and *Neisseria gonorrhoeae*. They are also useful in treating certain of the agents that cause atypical pneumonia such as *Coxiella burnetii* and *Chlamydia psittaci* and in the treatment of staphylococcal and streptococcal infections, depending on local resistance patterns. These agents should not be used in pregnancy.

β-lactamase test

There are several ways of determining if bacteria produce β-lactamase. These are based on the use of the chromogenic cephalosporin nitrocefin. The compound has a pale yellow colour, but when the amide bond of the β-lactam ring is cleaved by the enzyme, the resulting conformation change in the molecule renders it red. The BBL Cefinase™ test consists of cellulose discs impregnated with Nitrocefin. A loop is dipped into a colony and rubbed on the disc in a manner similar to the oxidase test (**70**). The appearance of a red colour indicates the isolate is β-lactamase-positive.

Allergies to antibiotics

Allergies to drugs are not uncommon and it is always important to ascertain any previous drug reactions that a patient may have had. Antibiotics are no exception, and in a few patients, allergic reactions to antibiotics can significantly limit the choice available to treat an infection.

Allergies to penicillin and other β-lactams are regularly reported. Penicillin itself is not antigenic, and does not initiate an immune response. However, degradation products of penicillin such as benzylpenicilloyl can covalently bind to human proteins. The penicilloyl residue is then converted to an antigenic determinant or hapten, and antibodies specific to this can be produced (**115**). On subsequent exposure to penicillin and related agents, an immunologically-mediated reaction can occur, which on occasion can be life-threatening.

Reactions can be classed as follows:
- Immediate. The reaction occurs within 30 minutes. This is characterized by urticaria, wheezing, hypotension, and shock. This reaction is due to IgE-mediated release of histamine from mast cells and basophils.
- Accelerated. The reaction occurs 1–72 hours after exposure. In addition to erythema, urticaria and wheezing, laryngeal oedema is a feature. IgE antibodies mediate this situation, but IgG antibodies are also involved.
- Late. This occurs 72 hours after exposure. A morbilliform (measles-like) skin rash with urticaria is characteristic. The mechanism is unclear.

An allergic reaction to penicillin implies a cross-reaction with other β-lactams including ampicillin, flucloxacillin, and the carbapenems. There is about a 5–10% chance of cross-reaction with the cephalosporins.

Comment

It is important to note that the information in this chapter is of a general nature. To use antibiotics correctly, the local antibiotic guidelines for a hospital or community must be referred to, as these give advice that is influenced by local practice and conditions. In all complicated cases the medical microbiologist or infectious diseases physician should be contacted to discuss antibiotic prescription.

It is now worthwhile to re-examine the diagrams showing the spectrum of activity of individual antibiotics, and to select antibiotics that would be needed in particular clinical settings to cover likely bacteria. For example, in the patient admitted from the community with an infection arising from an abdominal source, cefuroxime and metronidazole could be used initially. Another option could be amoxicillin, plus gentamicin and metronidazole. For the patient with an immediate allergic reaction to penicillin, and with renal failure, vancomycin plus ciprofloxacin and metronidazole could be one combination. Remembering the spectrum of activity of individual antibiotics and combination options will help in correct antibiotic prescription.

The resistance of a bacterium to antibiotics, the mechanisms involved, and laboratory methods for investigating resistance are a vast subject of their own. General textbooks cover this in some detail. Texts that are particularly useful include Mandell, Douglas, and Bennett's *Principle and Practice of Infectious Diseases*. The sixth edition of this book was published in 2004. In addition to comprehensive chapters on antibiotics, each clinical section covers practical antibiotic use. Such a text should be found in the medical school library. A recent review (Chan C, Livermore D [2004]. *Unmasking Antibacterial Resistance*. Merck & Co), gives a useful overview of resistance mechanisms. The British National Formulary is one example of a national document on all medical agents and should be referred to for indications, dosage, side-effects, and interactions of antibiotics.

With the continuing problem of antibiotic resistance, new agents are being produced. These include agents such as linezolid, an oxazolidinone, and pristinamycin, which have useful activity against a wide range of gram-positive bacteria. With the increasing importance of ESBL producing 'coliforms', the carbapenems are central to treatment here (Shah PM, Isaacs RD [2003)] Ertapenem, the first of a new group of carbapenems. *Journal of Antimicrobial Chemotherapy*, **52:** 538–542).

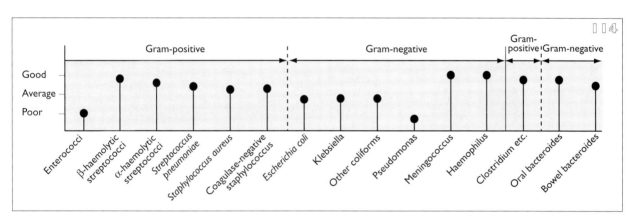

114 The range of activity of chloramphenicol.

115 Penicillin derivatives on their own are not allergens. However, upon binding to host proteins it is recognized as an antigen or hapten, and specific antibodies are produced to the hapten.

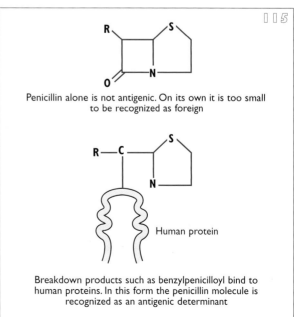

Penicillin alone is not antigenic. On its own it is too small to be recognized as foreign

Breakdown products such as benzylpenicilloyl bind to human proteins. In this form the penicillin molecule is recognized as an antigenic determinant

5 Infections of the Blood: Bacteraemia and Endocarditis

Introduction

Bacteraemia defines the presence of bacteria in the blood as detected by blood culture. Septicaemia also defines the presence of bacteria in blood, but it signals a sense of urgency in the management of the patient. The terms sepsis and septic shock are also used and, with clinical parameters such as fever, hypotension, tachycardia, leukophilia, and multi-organ failure, they define the severity of the situation.

A bacteraemia can be defined as transient (a single episode lasting less than 20 minutes), intermittent, or continuous (**116a–c**). These definitions are important concepts in terms of the site from which they may arise. An intermittent bacteraemia implies the manipulation of an extravascular site, such as a *Staphylococcus aureus* abscess, where bacteria enter the lymphatics at various times, and from there, the blood. A continuous

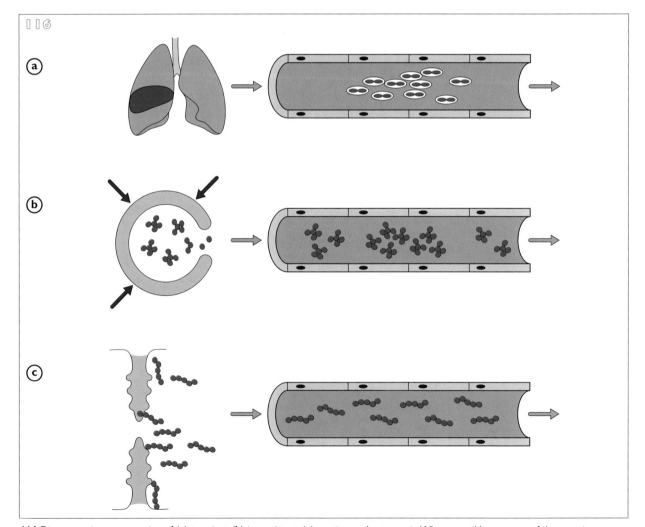

116 Diagrammatic representation of (**a**) transient, (**b**) intermittent, (**c**) continuous bacteraemia. Where possible, a source of the organism should be identified.

bacteraemia implies an intravascular source, and endocarditis is the most important example.

The presence of a few bacteria in the blood for short periods of time is likely to be a common event. For example, it is recognized that manipulation of teeth, including brushing, enables small numbers of oral bacteria to enter the blood. The presence of these few organisms is usually of no consequence as the natural defences rapidly clear them. Even when recognized pathogens enter the blood, their effect on the host may not be serious. On occasion, the medical microbiologist may telephone the result of a positive blood culture to a clinician to find that the patient, admitted the day before, has been discharged home without antibiotics. The blood culture, taken on admission contains for example, gram-positive diplococci, subsequently identified as pneumococcus. Here, rapid clearance of the organisms from the blood resolved the situation. It is reasonable to assume that individuals in the community who are 'unwell' for a short period of time may have pathogenic organisms in the blood, but the natural defences clear them. If these defences fail, the individual is more likely to seek medical advice.

Once bacteria enter the blood, they have the potential to settle in other sites of the body, and set up another focus of infection. A pneumococcal bacteraemia, arising from the lung, may result in bacteria settling on a heart valve to initiate acute bacterial endocarditis, or they may cross the blood–brain barrier to initiate meningitis. The bacteria may also cross the synovial membrane of a joint to initiate acute septic arthritis. These examples emphasize the importance of a full anatomical assessment of the bacteraemic or septic patient.

An important defence system of the blood is the macrophage population of the spleen and also the liver. It is recognized that individuals who have had a splenectomy are at risk of overwhelming infection with encapsulated bacteria such as pneumococcus and meningococcus. One reason for this is that the phagocytic function of the splenic macrophages is absent in these patients.

Organisms

Some examples of sources of bacteraemias and the organisms involved are shown in **117**. In the case of meningococcal sepsis, one organism is relevant. In the setting of bacteraemia arising from a bowel source, such as

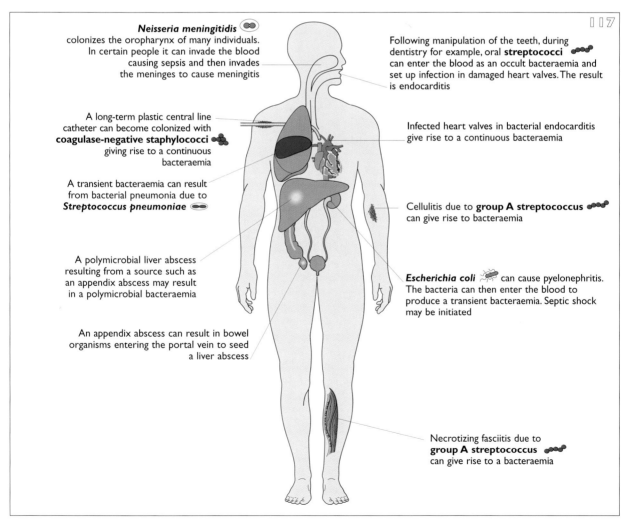

Neisseria meningitidis colonizes the oropharynx of many individuals. In certain people it can invade the blood causing sepsis and then invades the meninges to cause meningitis

A long-term plastic central line catheter can become colonized with **coagulase-negative staphylococci** giving rise to a continuous bacteraemia

A transient bacteraemia can result from bacterial pneumonia due to *Streptococcus pneumoniae*

A polymicrobial liver abscess resulting from a source such as an appendix abscess may result in a polymicrobial bacteraemia

An appendix abscess can result in bowel organisms entering the portal vein to seed a liver abscess

Following manipulation of the teeth, during dentistry for example, oral **streptococci** can enter the blood as an occult bacteraemia and set up infection in damaged heart valves. The result is endocarditis

Infected heart valves in bacterial endocarditis give rise to a continuous bacteraemia

Cellulitis due to **group A streptococcus** can give rise to bacteraemia

Escherichia coli can cause pyelonephritis. The bacteria can then enter the blood to produce a transient bacteraemia. Septic shock may be initiated

Necrotizing fasciitis due to **group A streptococcus** can give rise to a bacteraemia

117 Some examples of the sources of transient, intermittent or continuous bacteraemias.

a diverticular abscess, any of the bacteria making up the bowel flora may be involved, including streptococci, enterococci, coliforms and anaerobes.

For the patient with suspected endocarditis, gram-positive bacteria are the most common organisms. Native valve subacute endocarditis is likely to be caused by the oral 'viridans' streptococci such as *Streptococcus mitis*. Acute endocarditis, for example in the intravenous drug user (IVDU), may be caused by streptococci of the *Streptococcus anginosus* group or *Staphylococcus aureus*. Prosthetic valve endocarditis (PVE) is usually caused by the coagulase-negative staphylococci, especially in the first year following valve replacement.

Pathogenesis

It is important to reconsider the pathogenic potential of bacteria in the situation of bacteraemia and sepsis. When *Neisseria meningitidis* crosses the epithelial layer of the oropharynx and enters the blood, it can initiate sepsis and septic shock within hours. If medical intervention, including antibiotics, is not given promptly, death can follow in a short period of time. On the other hand, the relatively non-pathogenic oral streptococci can settle on an anatomically abnormal heart valve following an occult bacteraemia during dental treatment. The resultant endocarditis, giving rise to a continuous bacteraemia, may only be noted weeks later when the patient complains of symptoms such as malaise, weight loss, and a low-grade fever. Blood tests may reveal anaemia, low albumin, and raised ESR and CRP, all markers of the chronic cytokine response arising from the infection.

The coagulase-negative staphylococci, which are ubiquitous skin organisms, can colonize foreign bodies such as long-term indwelling intravenous catheters. In patients with long-term central venous lines, such colonization can result in an intermittent or continuous bacteraemia. The morbidity associated with this, characterized by a swinging fever, and the extensive use of antibiotics such as the glycopeptides make this an important problem.

Bacterial endocarditis
Native valve endocarditis

In native valve endocarditis there is usually some predisposing anatomical abnormality of the affected valve. These defects may be congenital or they may arise as a result of acquired conditions such as rheumatic fever or, more commonly nowadays, degenerative valve disease of ageing. As the flow of blood through the valve orifice is abnormal, the resulting turbulence can damage the valve endothelium. Fibrin and platelets are deposited on the damaged surface and such deposits can be colonized by bacteria passing through the valve orifice. The process is outlined in **118** and **119**. With the IVDU, it is possible that particulate contaminants in the injected material directly damage the valve endothelium. Fibrin and platelets are then deposited.

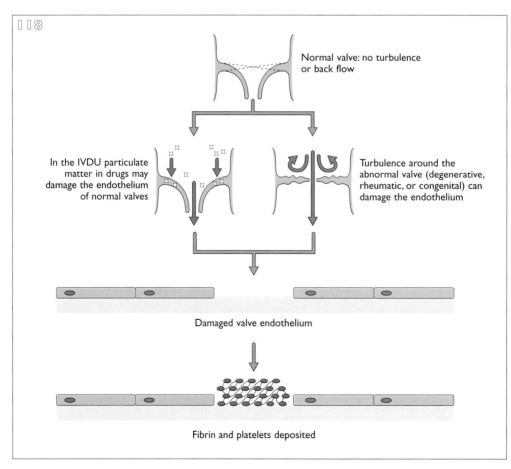

118

Normal valve: no turbulence or back flow

In the IVDU particulate matter in drugs may damage the endothelium of normal valves

Turbulence around the abnormal valve (degenerative, rheumatic, or congenital) can damage the endothelium

Damaged valve endothelium

Fibrin and platelets deposited

118 An outline of the pathological changes that occur in heart valves that predispose to bacterial endocarditis. (IVDU: intravenous drug user.)

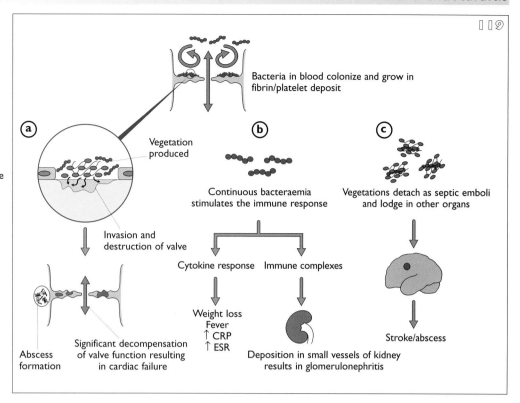

119 Bacteria from an occult bacteraemia initiate endocarditis. (**a**) Destruction of the valve can occur. (**b**) The continuous bacteraemia stimulates the immune system. (**c**) Vegetations can detach from the infected valve, and the resultant emboli can lodge in distant organs. (CRP: C-reactive protein; ESR: erythrocyte sedimentation rate.)

Once the bacteria have established a niche, their reproduction can lead to localized valve damage and the formation of vegetation. The damage can progress to gross compromise of valve function with resulting heart failure. Abscess formation in the valve root and spread of the infection into the myocardium can occur (**119a**). The continuous bacteraemia arising from the infected valve stimulates the immune system. The chronic cytokine response results in weight loss and fever, and immune complexes deposited in the kidney can cause glomerulonephritis (**119b**). Infected emboli from the vegetation can lodge in the arterial system of any organ. For example, septic emboli in the brain can produce a stroke (**119c**).

Although frowned upon by some, the terms 'acute' and 'subacute' endocarditis are still used, and indicate a degree of severity of the condition. The patient with subacute endocarditis may present with symptoms of weight loss and fever of weeks duration, and positive blood cultures confirm the diagnosis. In acute endocarditis there may be rapid compromise of cardiac function, secondary to a failing valve.

Prosthetic valve endocarditis

A prosthetic valve will create local abnormalities in blood flow and turbulence may damage the endothelium adjacent to the valve. Deposition of fibrin and platelets will give rise to a structure that can be colonized by bacteria (**120**). PVE is divided into early and late endocarditis. Early PVE occurs within 1 year of valve replacement and is often caused by coagulase-negative staphylococci introduced at the time of operation. As these are relatively non-pathogenic bacteria, the symptoms and signs of infection are often similar to subacute endocarditis discussed above. Late endocarditis is defined as that occurring 1 year after valve replacement and

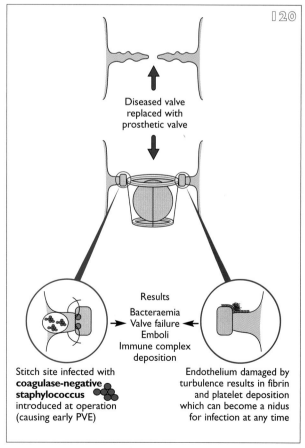

120 Replacement of a native valve with a prosthetic valve can predispose to prosthetic valve endocarditis (PVE). Bacteria such as the coagulase-negative staphylococci are important.

can be caused by a wide range of bacteria and fungi. The diagnosis of PVE must be considered promptly in any unwell patient with a prosthetic valve. Blood cultures are the cornerstone of diagnosis. Conservative treatment with antibiotics may be successful; however, replacement of the prosthetic valve is not infrequent.

Diagnosis

Blood culture is central to the management of the bacteraemic and/or septic patient. It is reasonable to collect one set of blood cultures in most cases but in the setting of bacterial endocarditis, 3–4 sets should be taken over a period of minutes or hours. This is to ensure that a continuous bacteraemia by one organism is identified, so that the type and length of antibiotic treatment can be clearly defined.

It is essential that the correct precautions are taken when collecting blood (**121**). If the skin over the usual collecting site on the antecubital fossa of the arm is not carefully cleaned with alcohol wipes, the blood taken can often be contaminated with the coagulase-negative staphylococci of the patient's skin or that of the blood taker. Blood cultures that grow these skin bacteria cloud any diagnosis, and are a waste of laboratory resources.

With a transient bacteraemia there is only a short period when the bacteria are in the blood before they are cleared by the body's defences. It is important to note that when blood is sampled, the number of bacteria present is usually in the order of about 10/mL of blood. Thus for adult patients about 5–10 mL of blood should be inoculated into both the aerobic and anaerobic blood culture bottles.

After inoculation with the patient's blood, blood culture bottles need to be promptly incubated at 37°C so that the bacteria can reproduce under optimal conditions. The blood culture bottle medium contains a rich basic medium and with the nutrients from the added blood itself, suitable conditions for growing most bacteria (and yeasts) are present.

In all modern bacteriology laboratories, blood culture bottles are placed in a blood culture machine. These machines have some automated system that regularly monitors for the presence of a reproducing bacterial population in each bottle. Some systems rely on detection of CO_2 gas produced during growth of the bacteria. The CO_2 appearing in the gas phase and being detected by a sensor is shown in **122**. Other systems use the following reaction taking place in the liquid phase of the blood culture bottle:

$$CO_2 + H_2O \rightarrow H_2CO_3 \rightarrow H^+ + HCO_3^-$$

A sensor system detects the increase in hydrogen ions, and a signal identifies the bottle as positive. In most cases a blood culture bottle becomes positive 24–48 hours after inoculation if there is a relevant organism present. When the machine registers a bottle as being positive, a portion of liquid from the bottle is removed for gram staining and various solid media, including sensitivity testing agar, are inoculated (**122**). Photomicrographs of examples of positive blood cultures are shown in **123a–c**.

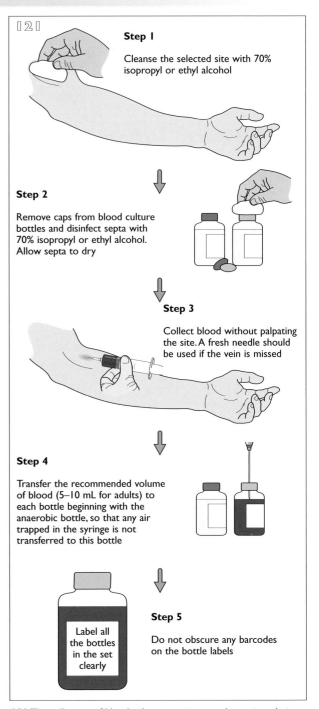

Step 1

Cleanse the selected site with 70% isopropyl or ethyl alcohol

Step 2

Remove caps from blood culture bottles and disinfect septa with 70% isopropyl or ethyl alcohol. Allow septa to dry

Step 3

Collect blood without palpating the site. A fresh needle should be used if the vein is missed

Step 4

Transfer the recommended volume of blood (5–10 mL for adults) to each bottle beginning with the anaerobic bottle, so that any air trapped in the syringe is not transferred to this bottle

Label all the bottles in the set clearly

Step 5

Do not obscure any barcodes on the bottle labels

121 The collection of blood cultures requires good aseptic technique in order to reduce the chance of contamination.

122 Inoculated blood culture bottles are incubated at 37°C to optimize growth of the bacteria. Positive bottles are removed from the blood culture machine, a sample of the liquid is removed, gram stained and plated directly onto culture and sensitivity testing agar.

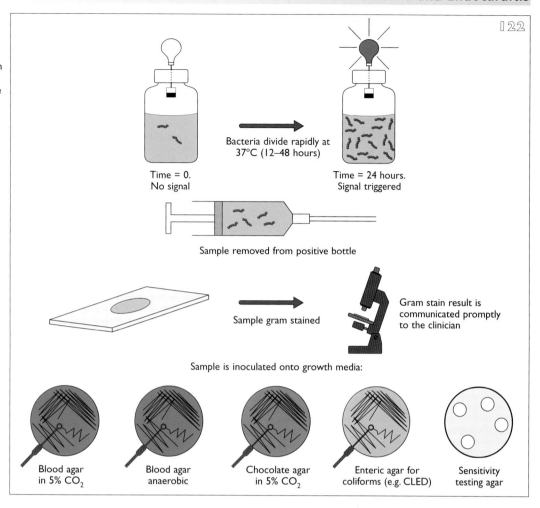

Time = 0.
No signal

Bacteria divide rapidly at 37°C (12–48 hours)

Time = 24 hours.
Signal triggered

Sample removed from positive bottle

Sample gram stained

Gram stain result is communicated promptly to the clinician

Sample is inoculated onto growth media:

Blood agar in 5% CO_2

Blood agar anaerobic

Chocolate agar in 5% CO_2

Enteric agar for coliforms (e.g. CLED)

Sensitivity testing agar

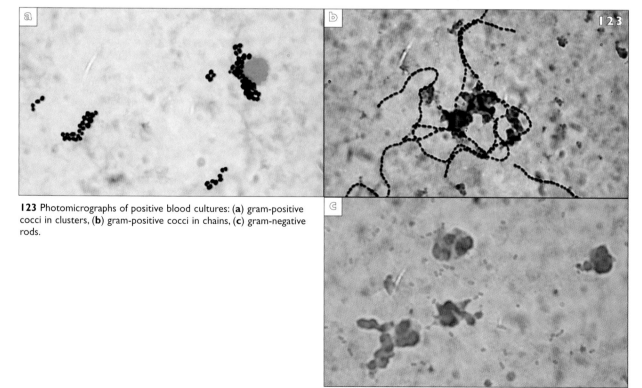

123 Photomicrographs of positive blood cultures: (**a**) gram-positive cocci in clusters, (**b**) gram-positive cocci in chains, (**c**) gram-negative rods.

The gram stain result is communicated to the clinician and a decision made regarding antibiotic prescription. The gram stain result also influences the antibiotics that are tested at this stage. For example, gram-positive bacteria would be tested against penicillin, amoxycillin, flucloxacillin, erythromycin, and vancomycin. Gram-negative bacteria would always be tested against an aminoglycoside such as gentamicin and β-lactams such as amoxycillin, co-amoxiclav, and cefuroxime. After overnight incubation of the agar plates the organism can be identified and its antibiotic susceptibility profile reported. Any unusual resistance profile needs to be discussed with the clinician and infection control team (ICT).

Examples of gram stain results of positive blood cultures in particular clinical settings are shown in **124**. The first gram-negative example here is useful. A patient is admitted with a UTI and possible pyelonephritis. Both blood culture and urine are collected. The urine would be processed promptly and plated onto media for identification and sensitivity testing, with results usually available the next day. When the blood culture is registered positive 24 hours or so after admission and shows gram-negative rods, the organism in the blood should be the same as that in the urine. If the patient is not improving, the antibiotic sensitivity result of the urine isolate must be used to modify the antibiotics being given to the patient.

Bacterial endocarditis
Culture-positive endocarditis
In an emergency situation associated with acute endocarditis, 2–3 sets of blood cultures should be collected over a period of about 20 minutes, and a high dose intravenous antibiotic regimen instituted, which must cover *Staphylococcus aureus*. The patient needs to be referred to the cardiologist and cardiothoracic surgeon. With subacute endocarditis, blood cultures are usually collected over several hours before an appropriate regime of antibiotics is prescribed. Three to four sets should be collected so that the relevance of any isolate

Gram stain	Patient	Other specimen?
Gram-positive diplococci	50-year-old male smoker with lobar pneumonia Most likely organism = *Streptococcus pneumoniae*	Purulent sputum taken on admission, growing pure growth of presumptive *Streptococcus pneumoniae*
Gram-positive cocci in clusters	25-year-old IVDU with symptoms and signs of endocarditis Most likely organism = *Staphylococcus aureus*	Abscess in groin drained on admission, growing **coagulase-positive staphylococcus**
Gram-positive cocci in clusters	25-year-old female with cystitis and ? pyelonephritis Most likely organism = **coagulase-negative staphylococcus** = contamination of blood culture by skin flora at time of collection	Purulent urine collected on admission, already grown pure growth of a **coliform**
Gram-positive cocci in clusters	69-year-old female with malaise and fever 7 weeks after insertion of prosthetic heart valve for degenerative valve disease. ? Endocarditis Most likely organism = **coagulase-negative staphylococcus** possibly causing PVE	None yet but 3–4 more sets of blood cultures must be collected before antibiotics are started
Gram-positive cocci in chains	32-year-old female who is pyrexial 2 days post-partum. Inflamed caesarian section wound and tender uterus Most likely organism = **group A streptococcus**, must consider necrotizing fasciitis here	None yet but appropriate wound and high vaginal swabs should be collected
Gram-negative rods	25-year-old female with cystitis and pyelonephritis Most likely organism = *Escherichia coli*	Purulent urine collected at admission, already grown a pure growth of a **coliform**
Gram-negative rods	25-year-old male returned 10 days ago from Pakistan, complaining of fever, abdominal tenderness, headache. ? Typhoid fever Most likely organism = *Salmonella typhi*	Stool specimens should be sent to the microbiology laboratory
Gram-negative diplococci	25-year-old female with meningitis and purpuric rash. ? Meningococcal sepsis and meningitis Most likely organism = *Neisseria meningitidis*	CSF collected on admission, no organisms seen on gram stain but culture growing presumptive *Neisseria meningitidis*

124 Examples of positive blood culture gram stain results, and the likely source of these bacteria. (CSF: cerebrospinal fluid; IVDU: intravenous drug user; PVE: prosthetic valve endocarditis.)

can be assessed. The example in **125** shows 7/8 bottles becoming positive within 48 hours of collection, and gram staining shows all these positive bottles growing gram-positive cocci in chains. The organism here is identified as *Streptococcus mutans*, a member of the oral flora. In the correct clinical setting this is clearly the organism causing the endocarditis. If only 1/8 or 2/8 bottles grew a streptococcus over a period of days, the relevance of the isolate may be doubted.

Culture-negative endocarditis

Not infrequently a patient may have the symptoms and signs of endocarditis, which are supported by laboratory results such as a raised ESR and CRP. However, all blood cultures are negative. The most common reason for culture-negative endocarditis is the recent use of antibiotics by the patient. These may render the blood 'sterile' for days. This highlights the importance of withholding antibiotics in the patient with suspected endocarditis until blood cultures have been taken.

It is also appropriate to consider a wider range of organisms when cultures are negative, and the medical microbiologist should be consulted. Organisms that may be considered are uncommon gram-negative bacteria such as cardiobacterium and kingella, which belong to the HACEK group, as well as 'atypical organisms' such as legionella and chlamydia (**126**).

Molecular diagnostic methods: the polymerase chain reaction

The PCR has become very useful for the diagnosis of meningococcal sepsis and meningitis. In cases of suspected meningococcal disease, a specimen of blood should also be collected in an EDTA tube. A sample of the specimen is then analysed by PCR; if meningococcus is present, specific sequences of meningococcal DNA will be amplified into a detectable signal. Because of the sensitivity of the method, results can be positive when blood cultures are negative. A current PCR enables the identification of the serogroup of *Neisseria meningitidis*.

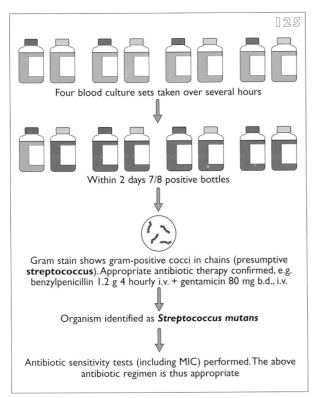

Four blood culture sets taken over several hours

↓

Within 2 days 7/8 positive bottles

↓

Gram stain shows gram-positive cocci in chains (presumptive **streptococcus**). Appropriate antibiotic therapy confirmed, e.g. benzylpenicillin 1.2 g 4 hourly i.v. + gentamicin 80 mg b.d., i.v.

↓

Organism identified as **Streptococcus mutans**

↓

Antibiotic sensitivity tests (including MIC) performed. The above antibiotic regimen is thus appropriate

125 An outline of the bacteriological management of subacute endocarditis. The standard antibiotic regimen instituted may be influenced by subsequent susceptibility profiles. The colour change in the positive bottles is for diagrammatic purposes only.

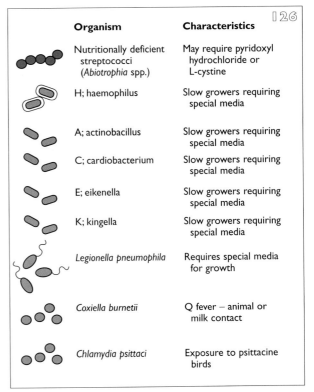

Organism	Characteristics
Nutritionally deficient streptococci (*Abiotrophia* spp.)	May require pyridoxyl hydrochloride or L-cystine
H; haemophilus	Slow growers requiring special media
A; actinobacillus	Slow growers requiring special media
C; cardiobacterium	Slow growers requiring special media
E; eikenella	Slow growers requiring special media
K; kingella	Slow growers requiring special media
Legionella pneumophila	Requires special media for growth
Coxiella burnetii	Q fever – animal or milk contact
Chlamydia psittaci	Exposure to psittacine birds

126 Organisms shown here should be considered in the setting of culture-negative endocarditis.

Treatment

When the clinically infected or septic patient has been assessed and specimens collected for microbiological investigation, an appropriate antibiotic or antibiotic combination must be prescribed. Examples of such antibiotic regimens are shown in **127**. The regimen used must take into account whether or not the patient has a penicillin allergy. Results of renal function tests should be examined, as they are important in determining the frequency of administering the aminoglycosides and vancomycin. The patient needs to be referred to the relevant specialist team. The cardiologist and the cardiothoracic surgeon must see a patient with acute endocarditis. The general or orthopaedic surgeon must promptly assess the patient with a severe cellulitis that may progress to necrotizing fasciitis.

Some examples of the length and route of administration of antibiotics that would be appropriate in certain clinical settings are shown in **128**. Note that for examples 1, 2 and 4, suitable antibiotics are started on the clinical evidence available on the admission of the patient, and their use is confirmed when blood cultures are positive. In example 3, the differential diagnosis would include malaria and typhoid fever. Ciprofloxacin is started when the blood cultures grow gram-negative rods, essentially confirming the diagnosis of typhoid. Another important point to note in the setting of an uncomplicated bacteraemia, is that if the patient rapidly responds to treatment and is apyrexial, intravenous antibiotics can be changed to an oral regime. The length of antibiotic treatment should usually be between 1–2 weeks. However, in complicated cases such as infective endocarditis, treatment must continue for 2–6 weeks depending on the organism involved.

Treatment of endocarditis

Some examples of antibiotic regimens to consider in endocarditis are shown in **129**. For streptococci, a regime of benzylpenicillin (unless the patient is allergic to penicillin), and gentamicin is usually appropriate. Microbiology laboratories should determine the MIC of penicillin as this determines the length of therapy; the Etest™ is suitable here. The combination of penicillin and

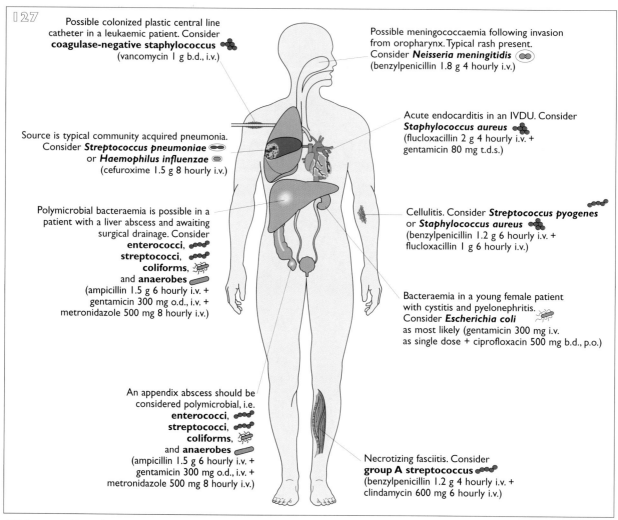

Possible colonized plastic central line catheter in a leukaemic patient. Consider **coagulase-negative staphylococcus** (vancomycin 1 g b.d., i.v.)

Possible meningococcaemia following invasion from oropharynx. Typical rash present. Consider *Neisseria meningitidis* (benzylpenicillin 1.8 g 4 hourly i.v.)

Source is typical community acquired pneumonia. Consider *Streptococcus pneumoniae* or *Haemophilus influenzae* (cefuroxime 1.5 g 8 hourly i.v.)

Acute endocarditis in an IVDU. Consider *Staphylococcus aureus* (flucloxacillin 2 g 4 hourly i.v. + gentamicin 80 mg t.d.s.)

Polymicrobial bacteraemia is possible in a patient with a liver abscess and awaiting surgical drainage. Consider **enterococci, streptococci, coliforms,** and **anaerobes** (ampicillin 1.5 g 6 hourly i.v. + gentamicin 300 mg o.d., i.v. + metronidazole 500 mg 8 hourly i.v.)

Cellulitis. Consider *Streptococcus pyogenes* or *Staphylococcus aureus* (benzylpenicillin 1.2 g 6 hourly i.v. + flucloxacillin 1 g 6 hourly i.v.)

Bacteraemia in a young female patient with cystitis and pyelonephritis. Consider *Escherichia coli* as most likely (gentamicin 300 mg i.v. as single dose + ciprofloxacin 500 mg b.d., p.o.)

An appendix abscess should be considered polymicrobial, i.e. **enterococci, streptococci, coliforms,** and **anaerobes** (ampicillin 1.5 g 6 hourly i.v. + gentamicin 300 mg o.d., i.v. + metronidazole 500 mg 8 hourly i.v.)

Necrotizing fasciitis. Consider **group A streptococcus** (benzylpenicillin 1.2 g 4 hourly i.v. + clindamycin 600 mg 6 hourly i.v.)

127 Some suitable antibiotics to consider in different clinical situations. Doses for a 60 kg adult patient with normal renal function.

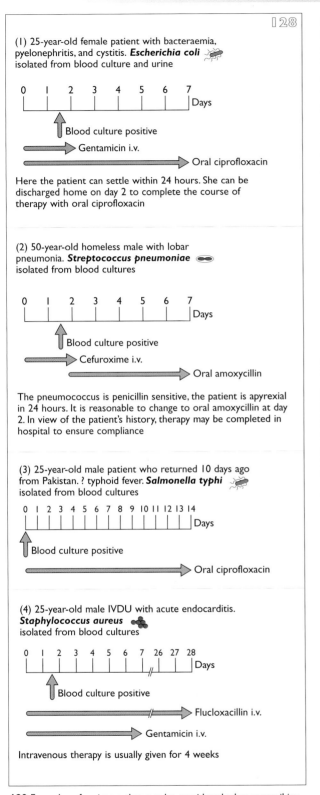

128 Examples of regimens that may be considered when prescribing antibiotics for various bacteraemias.

(1) 25-year-old female patient with bacteraemia, pyelonephritis, and cystitis. *Escherichia coli* isolated from blood culture and urine

Here the patient can settle within 24 hours. She can be discharged home on day 2 to complete the course of therapy with oral ciprofloxacin

(2) 50-year-old homeless male with lobar pneumonia. *Streptococcus pneumoniae* isolated from blood cultures

The pneumococcus is penicillin sensitive, the patient is apyrexial in 24 hours. It is reasonable to change to oral amoxycillin at day 2. In view of the patient's history, therapy may be completed in hospital to ensure compliance

(3) 25-year-old male patient who returned 10 days ago from Pakistan. ? typhoid fever. *Salmonella typhi* isolated from blood cultures

(4) 25-year-old male IVDU with acute endocarditis. *Staphylococcus aureus* isolated from blood cultures

Intravenous therapy is usually given for 4 weeks

129 Some examples of antibiotic regimens that are used in the treatment of infective endocarditis. Dose for a 60 kg adult patient with normal renal function. (PVE: prosthetic valve endocarditis.)

gentamicin acts synergistically, as the effect of the two agents together is greater than their separate additive effect. This synergy relies on penicillin damaging the cell wall sufficiently to allow the gentamicin to enter the cell and interfere with protein synthesis. On its own gentamicin would not be able to enter the streptococcal cell at the normal therapeutic concentrations used.

The enterococci tend to be more difficult organisms to treat, as they often exhibit tolerance to antibiotics. Ampicillin or amoxycillin are usually used instead of penicillin. A gentamicin Etest™ should be done; if the MIC is <100 mg/L, synergistic gentamicin can be used. Where the MIC is greater than this, 6 weeks of therapy with ampicillin or amoxycillin is needed and an alternative second agent such as streptomycin needs to be considered. Note that in treating streptococcal and enterococcal endocarditis, the 'pulse dose' aminoglycoside regimen is not regarded as being suitable, and for adults with normal renal function, gentamicin 80 mg b.d. is used in synergistic combination with penicillin, ampicillin, or amoxycillin. The glycopeptides vancomycin and teicoplanin replace β-lactams in the penicillin allergic patient.

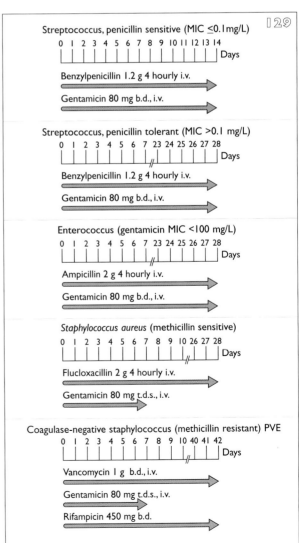

Response to treatment

Patients with endocarditis must be assessed regularly. It is also important to examine the temperature chart at least daily. Blood tests such as CRP and ESR should also be checked on a regular basis. The return of the temperature, CRP, and ESR to normal values after starting treatment is reassuring (**130a**). A spiking temperature that persists beyond 5–7 days must warrant reinvestigation of the patient for the possibility of a valve or myocardial abscess or septic embolus (**130b**). The example here is clearly exaggerated, but underlines the importance of using simple parameters in the management of the patient. Drug induced fevers should also be considered.

Septic shock

Septic shock is a term associated with recognized pathogens such as pneumococcus, meningococcus, group A streptococcus, and coliforms. However, in patients defined as being in septic shock, blood cultures are negative in at least 50% of cases. These patients are usually treated in ICU, where antibiotics are given empirically. It is important to recognize that the shock may also be due to the systemic inflammatory response and not the direct result of an invading organism or its toxins.

Any antibiotic regime in the intensive care setting thus needs to be reviewed regularly in the light of microbiology results and the clinical condition of the patient. Some of the interventions used to support the patient in intensive care are shown in **131**. Ventilation, the presence of arterial and venous lines, and a urinary catheter breach the natural defences of the body. The ICU patient is thus at risk of nosocomial infection as well, and ventilation-associated pneumonia and line infections are particular problems which need to be regularly monitored.

Prevention, prophylaxis and public health issues

Prevention

It is important to bear in mind that vaccination can prevent invasive disease such as bacteraemia and sepsis. The encapsulated bacteria, haemophilus, pneumococcus, and meningococcus, are examples where effective vaccines exist. The development of the *Haemophilus influenzae* type b (Hib) vaccine has largely eliminated invasive haemophilus infection in children less than 5 years of age in countries where this vaccination is practised. The older individual with chronic obstructive airways disease (COAD) should be vaccinated with the 23-valent-pneumococcal vaccine.

Splenectomized patients should receive the pneumococcal, meningococcal, and Hib vaccines. It is also recommended that these individuals take penicillin long term. In addition they should carry a medic alert bracelet or a warning card (**132**).

Public health issues

Two examples are considered here. The patient with confirmed or suspected typhoid fever or meningococcal septicaemia must be notified to the consultant in communicable disease control (CCDC) or public health doctor immediately.

It is the responsibility of these health care workers to identify possible routes of transmission of an organism, and to identify any 'at risk' individuals in the community. For example, it is essential that a patient with typhoid fever who is a food handler should not be allowed to return to this occupation until stool carriage of *Salmonella typhi* has been eliminated. A 2-week course of oral ciprofloxacin is usually effective.

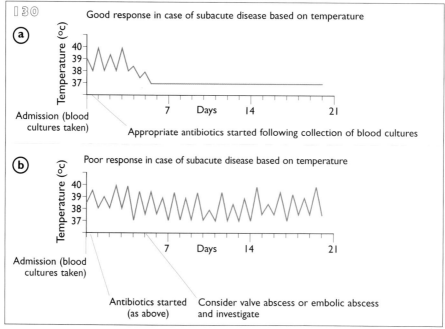

130 A simple parameter such as temperature monitoring is important in management of the patient with endocarditis. (**a**) A good response. (**b**) A poor response that clearly requires further investigation.

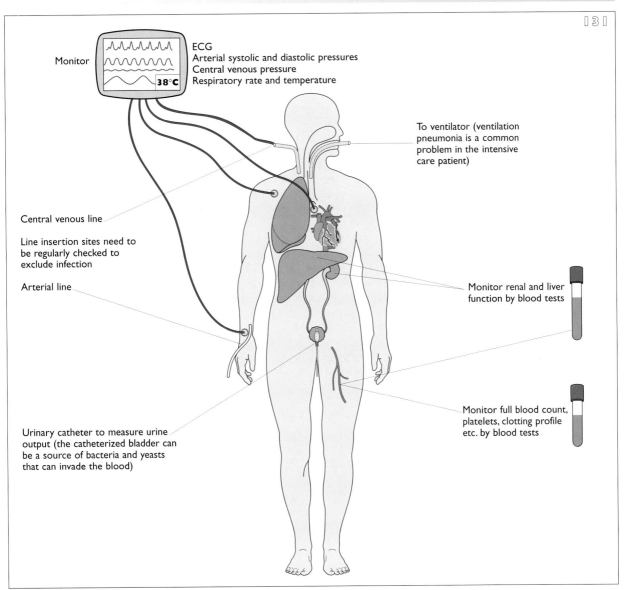

131 The intensive care patient is given ventilatory and cardiac support, and organ functions are monitored electronically and by biochemical and haematology tests. Interventions such as ventilation and catheters can predispose to nosocomial infection. (ECG: electrocardiogram)

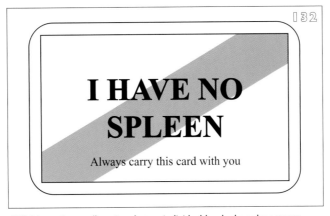

132 A 'warning card' stating that an individual has had a splenectomy should be carried.

In the case of a suspected or confirmed case of meningococcal sepsis and/or meningitis, the CCDC would identify possible contacts of the index case in the setting of the home, workplace, school, or university. Antibiotic prophylaxis such as RIF would then be given to the contacts. It is important to appreciate that prophylaxis is not primarily to prevent meningococcal infection in an individual, but to reduce the overall nasopharyngeal carriage rate in an 'at risk' population, thus minimizing the chance of invasive disease occurring. The identification of the menigococcal serotype causing disease is important, as vaccination of the index case and the identified contacts is important. For example, serotype B is more common in the United Kingdom. Vaccines for types A and C, but not B, are currently available.

Antibiotic prophylaxis to prevent endocarditis.

The patient who is at risk of endocarditis needs to be given appropriate prophylactic antibiotics for certain procedures in order to prevent either native valve endocarditis or PVE. Some of the procedures that may predispose to the development of endocarditis and suitable antibiotics to use are shown in **133**. Note that clindamycin should not be used 'below the diaphragm' as this agent has poor enterococcal activity. Enterococci are of importance in PVE.

The need for prophylaxis is identified when individuals have valve lesions, septal defects, a patent ductus, or prosthetic valve. Patients with a prosthetic valve or with a previous history of endocarditis are identified as at special risk, and the initial dose of the prophylactic antibiotics is usually given intravenously. It is important that patients with endocarditis have their teeth assessed by oral-facial surgeons, so that any sites of chronic infection can be identified and treated.

Comment

More details on sepsis and septic shock and the mechanisms involved can be found in general microbiology and infectious diseases textbooks. This is a rapidly advancing field as details of the interaction between microorganisms, cells of the immune system, cytokines, and coagulation pathways are unravelled by research. Out of this new treatment regimes are being developed.

A review in the *New England Journal of Medicine* highlights this:

Matthay M (2001). Severe sepsis – a new treatment with both anticoagulant and anti-inflammatory properties. *New England Journal of Medicine* **344**: 759–61.

More detailed information on the management of infective endocarditis can be found in general medical microbiology and infectious diseases textbooks. The chapters in Mandell, Douglas, and Bennett's *Principles and Practice of Infectious Diseases* are very good. More detailed information can be found in the following papers:

Guidelines of the Working Party of the British Society for Antimicrobial Chemotherapy (1998). Antibiotic treatment of streptococcal, enterococcal, and staphylococcal endocarditis. *HEART* **79**: 207–10.

Hoesley CJ, Cobbs CG (1999). Endocarditis at the millennium. *Journal of Infectious Diseases* **179**: 360–5.

Shanson DC (1998). New guidelines for the antibiotic treatment of streptococcal, enterococcal and staphylococcal endocarditis. *Journal of Antimicrobial Chemotherapy* **42**: 292–6.

The Hoesley and Cobbs reference provides a useful review and highlights the Duke criteria that should be used when there is any doubt about the diagnosis of a case of infective endocarditis. These criteria include clinical, laboratory, microbiology, and imaging parameters.

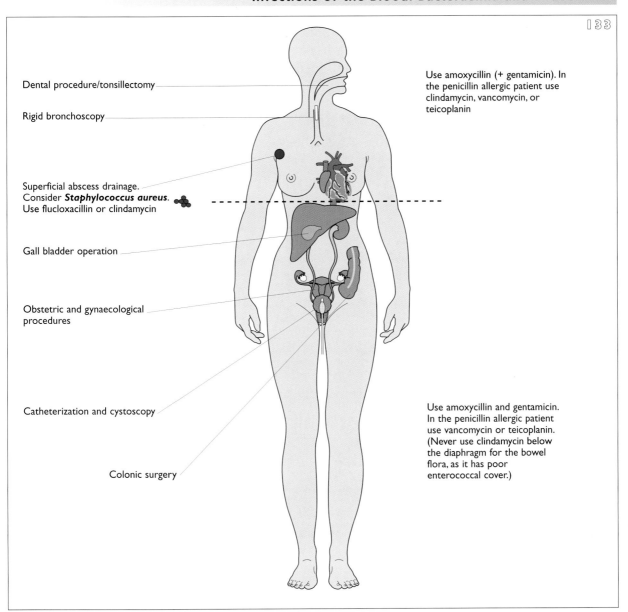

Dental procedure/tonsillectomy

Rigid bronchoscopy

Use amoxycillin (+ gentamicin). In the penicillin allergic patient use clindamycin, vancomycin, or teicoplanin

Superficial abscess drainage. Consider *Staphylococcus aureus*. Use flucloxacillin or clindamycin

Gall bladder operation

Obstetric and gynaecological procedures

Use amoxycillin and gentamicin. In the penicillin allergic patient use vancomycin or teicoplanin. (Never use clindamycin below the diaphragm for the bowel flora, as it has poor enterococcal cover.)

Catheterization and cystoscopy

Colonic surgery

133 Some examples of when antibiotic prophylaxis needs to be considered in the patient with a valve lesion, or other cardiac abnormality.

6 Infections of the Alimentary Canal

Introduction

Infections of the alimentary canal are a major cause of morbidity and mortality throughout the world. Millions of children under the age of 5 years die each year as a result of gastroenteritis. Bacteria, viruses (e.g. rotavirus), and protozoa (e.g. *Giardia lamblia* and *Entamoeba histolytica*) gain access to the gastrointestinal tract via the mouth. Often a water supply contaminated with human effluent is the source of these organisms, and large outbreaks of disease associated with crowding, such as that in refugee camps, occur. Contaminated food is an important source of organisms and outbreaks associated with the consumption of food at gatherings are regularly reported. Infections transmitted from animals, or zoonoses, are also relevant; for example *Escherichia coli* O157 can be transmitted directly from the normal intestinal flora of bovines to humans.

In developed parts of the world, campylobacter is the most common bacterial cause of gastroenteritis, followed by salmonella and shigella. In tropical and underdeveloped areas of the world, bacteria such as *Vibrio cholerae* also assume importance. In all cases of food poisoning, vomiting or diarrhoea, it is important to identify the possible source of infection and the mode of transmission (**134**). This is necessary if an outbreak in a family, school or community is to be controlled. A history of travel either within a country or to other parts of the world is important in determining the possible source of an infectious agent.

Gastrointestinal tract infections can also be acquired within hospitals. Antibiotic-associated diarrhoea is usually linked to the gram-positive anaerobe *Clostridium difficile*, and is a particular problem in the older hospitalized patient, in whom it can produce a life-threatening diarrhoeal illness. Perhaps the most unusual organism causing disease in the gastrointestinal tract is *Helicobacter pylori*. This bacterium can inhabit the inhospitable environment of the stomach and is a cause of gastric and duodenal ulcer disease, and malignancy.

The 'normal' bacterial flora of the alimentary canal can also cause disease. The oral streptococci and anaerobes of the mouth are the agents of dental caries and periodontal infection. The bacterial flora of the intestines is involved in appendix and diverticular abscesses and biliary tract sepsis; such infections often arise as a result of some anatomical abnormality.

The alimentary canal has its own natural defences based on normal anatomy and physiology. In addition, the normal bacterial flora is an essential part of the defence. This normal flora creates an environment in which

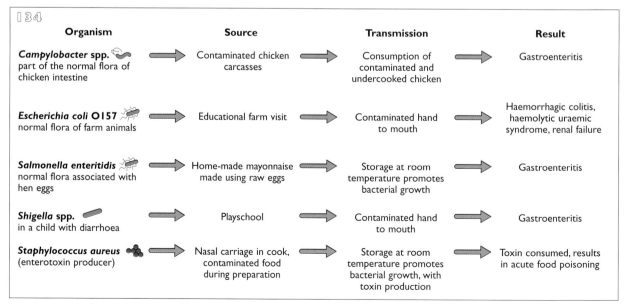

	Organism	Source	Transmission	Result
Campylobacter spp. part of the normal flora of chicken intestine		Contaminated chicken carcasses	Consumption of contaminated and undercooked chicken	Gastroenteritis
Escherichia coli O157 normal flora of farm animals		Educational farm visit	Contaminated hand to mouth	Haemorrhagic colitis, haemolytic uraemic syndrome, renal failure
Salmonella enteritidis normal flora associated with hen eggs		Home-made mayonnaise made using raw eggs	Storage at room temperature promotes bacterial growth	Gastroenteritis
Shigella spp. in a child with diarrhoea		Playschool	Contaminated hand to mouth	Gastroenteritis
Staphylococcus aureus (enterotoxin producer)		Nasal carriage in cook, contaminated food during preparation	Storage at room temperature promotes bacterial growth, with toxin production	Toxin consumed, results in acute food poisoning

134 Some examples of the source and mode of transmission of common bacterial causes of gastrointestinal infection in a developed country.

exogenous pathogens are less likely to establish themselves and initiate disease. Some examples of important defences of the alimentary canal are shown in **135**. The contents of the lumen, the structural integrity of the mucosal and submucosal layers of the bowel, and the bowel-associated lymphoid aggregates are three broad defences. As the colon is filled with bacteria, it is reasonable to assume that small numbers of these organisms can cross the mucosal lining and subsequently enter the portal vein where they are transported to the liver. Here macrophages, termed Kupffer cells, usually clear these bacteria from the blood. Some examples of how changes to the natural defences of the alimentary canal can predispose to infection are shown in **136**.

135 Normal anatomy, physiology, and a normal bacterial flora are essential defence mechanisms of the alimentary canal.

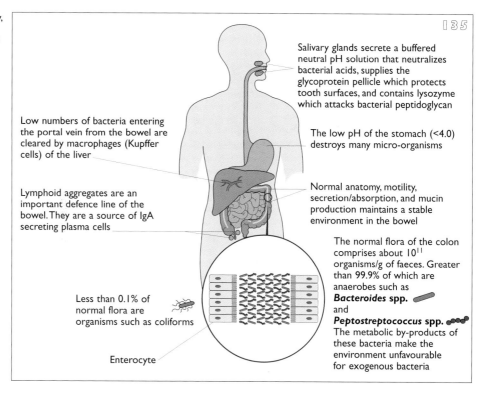

135

Salivary glands secrete a buffered neutral pH solution that neutralizes bacterial acids, supplies the glycoprotein pellicle which protects tooth surfaces, and contains lysozyme which attacks bacterial peptidoglycan

Low numbers of bacteria entering the portal vein from the bowel are cleared by macrophages (Kupffer cells) of the liver

The low pH of the stomach (<4.0) destroys many micro-organisms

Lymphoid aggregates are an important defence line of the bowel. They are a source of IgA secreting plasma cells

Normal anatomy, motility, secretion/absorption, and mucin production maintains a stable environment in the bowel

The normal flora of the colon comprises about 10^{11} organisms/g of faeces. Greater than 99.9% of which are anaerobes such as **Bacteroides spp.** and **Peptostreptococcus spp.** The metabolic by-products of these bacteria make the environment unfavourable for exogenous bacteria

Less than 0.1% of normal flora are organisms such as coliforms

Enterocyte

136 Any changes to the normal anatomy, physiology, and bacterial flora of the alimentary canal may predispose to infection.

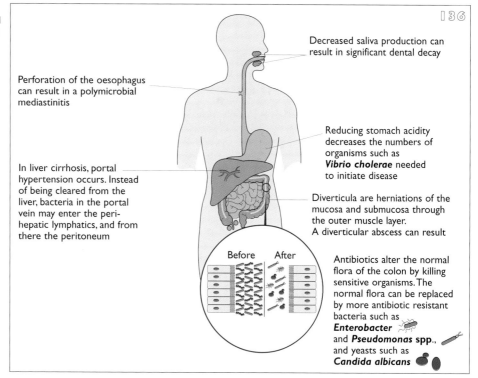

136

Decreased saliva production can result in significant dental decay

Perforation of the oesophagus can result in a polymicrobial mediastinitis

Reducing stomach acidity decreases the numbers of organisms such as **Vibrio cholerae** needed to initiate disease

In liver cirrhosis, portal hypertension occurs. Instead of being cleared from the liver, bacteria in the portal vein may enter the peri-hepatic lymphatics, and from there the peritoneum

Diverticula are herniations of the mucosa and submucosa through the outer muscle layer. A diverticular abscess can result

Before After

Antibiotics alter the normal flora of the colon by killing sensitive organisms. The normal flora can be replaced by more antibiotic resistant bacteria such as **Enterobacter** and **Pseudomonas spp.**, and yeasts such as **Candida albicans**

Organisms

The bacteria that cause disease in the alimentary canal can be divided into exogenous and endogenous (**137**). Food and water are the usual sources of exogenous bacteria, but *Clostridium difficile* can be acquired from the hospital environment, where it survives as a heat-stable spore. *Helicobacter pylori* is likely to be spread from human to human via the oral–oral and faecal–oral routes. In the case of enterotoxigenic *Staphylococcus aureus* and *Bacillus cereus*,

the organisms multiply in contaminated food that is stored incorrectly, for example at room temperature rather than in a fridge. The bacteria secrete toxins, and when the food is consumed, nausea and vomiting occur 1–6 hours later.

Endogenous bacteria are the agents of dental and gingival disease of the mouth. The streptococci, enterococci, coliforms, and anaerobes of the intestines are those to consider in any infection of the bowel such as an appendix, liver, or diverticular abscess.

137 A list of bacteria which should be considered in infective conditions of the alimentary canal. For exogenous bacteria the main mechanism of disease is indicated (In: invasion; Inf: inflammation; P: penetration; T: toxin).

Pathogenesis
Dental infections

Bacteria making up the normal flora of the mouth colonize particular parts of the tooth and gingival surface (**138**). The acid metabolic by-products of these bacteria, arising from the fermentation of dietary sugar, are important causes of tooth decay. Teeth are protected by the cleaning action of the tongue, the buffering effect of saliva and the acquired pellicle, derived from saliva, which coats the surface of teeth. This coating, which becomes colonized with bacteria, is removed by regular cleaning and is then replaced by new pellicle, thus preventing decay (**139a**). In the setting of poor oral hygiene, where for example crevices are not cleaned properly, a nidus of infection may arise, with the development of dental caries (**139b**). The infection can progress to pulpitis and apical abscess formation (**139c**). Infection of the gums begins as subgingival plaque, progressing to periodontitis. The anaerobes of the mouth are important here (**139d**).

138 The cross section of a tooth. Certain bacteria of the normal mouth flora occupy certain ecological niches around the tooth and have the potential to cause dental infection.

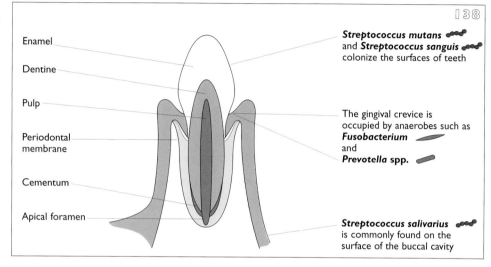

139 (**a**) Tooth cleaning removes the pellicle and associated bacteria. (**b**) If bacteria are not removed they initiate decay. (**c**) The decay can progress to pulpitis and alveolar abscess. (**d**) Periodontal disease leads to periodontitis and abscess formation.

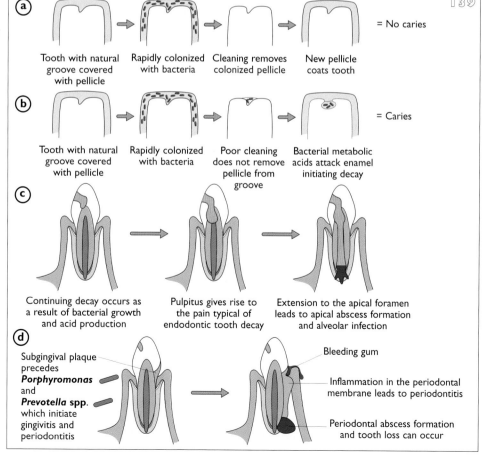

Infections of the teeth can spread into adjacent bone to initiate osteomyelitis, can cause local soft tissue abscess, and have the potential to spread to the facial sinuses. In the setting of widespread tooth decay, aspiration of the mouth flora may result in the development of a lung abscess. Profound halitosis may be present, indicating that the oral anaerobes are growing in the lung! Some local and distant sites where the consequences of tooth decay can manifest are shown in **140**.

Infections of the upper gastrointestinal tract
Endogenous organisms
Perforation of the oesophagus may arise for several reasons and the result is often a polymicrobial mediastinitis. Dilators used to alleviate dysphagia in the patient with carcinoma of the oesophagus or endoscopes used in gastroscopy can cause perforation. Vomiting, associated with sudden pressure changes, can also result in tearing of the lower end of the oesophagus (Boerhaave's syndrome). Perforation of the duodenum as a result of ulcer disease can result in spillage of organisms into the peritoneum.

Exogenous organisms
Helicobacter pylori may reside in the inhospitable acid environment of the stomach for months or years before clinical disease is noted, colonizing gastric-type epithelial cells in the stomach and duodenum. Pathogenic properties of the organism and some features of infection are shown in **141a, b**. The motility of the bacterium enables it to reside in the mucin layer and NH_3, produced by a potent urease, neutralizes the acid of the stomach. Adhesion, a cytotoxin, the toxic effect of ammonia, and the strong inflammatory response lead to gastritis and then peptic and duodenal ulceration. The long-term consequences of the infection can be gastric malignancies such as adenocarcinoma and lymphoma.

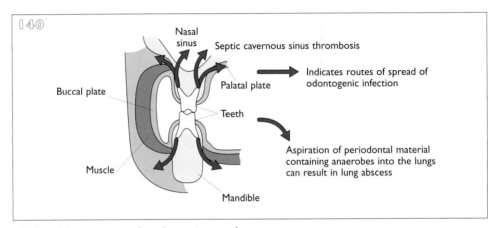

140 Dental disease can spread to adjacent tissues and organs.

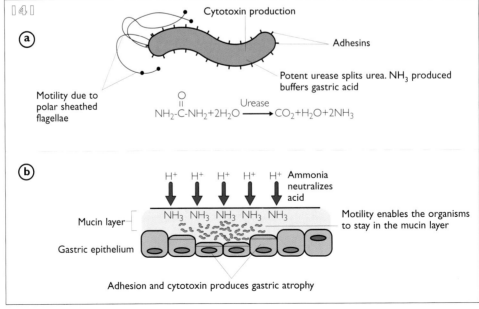

141 (**a**) Some of the pathogenic properties of *Helicobacter pylori*. (**b**) Some features of the mechanism of helicobacter infection.

Infections of the lower gastrointestinal tract
Exogenous organisms

In order to cause disease here, pathogens such as shigella, salmonella and *Vibrio cholerae* have to traverse the inhospitable lumen of the stomach. There are significant differences in the infecting dose of these bacteria, being about 10^2, 10^5 and 10^8 organisms/dose respectively. Illness arising from these organisms usually manifests 24–48 hours after the contaminated food or water is ingested.

There are three broad mechanisms whereby bacteria cause gastroenteritis. These are interference with the secretory and absorptive properties of the intestine by adherence and/or enterotoxin, invasion of the mucosal enterocytes, or penetration of organisms through the mucosa, where they multiply in cells of the bowel-associated lymphoid tissue.

An important process contributing to diarrhoea is loss of the enterocyte microvilli. This effacement, caused by adherence of the bacteria, alters the secretory and absorptive properties of the enterocyte, disturbing the normal water and electrolyte balance of the small intestine (**142a**). Enteroadhesive *Escherichia coli* is an example, but it is likely that most of the bacteria discussed here will bring about some degree of effacement in the course of their interaction with the surface of the enterocyte. *Vibrio cholerae*, for example, binds to the microvilli causing effacement, but it is the A component of the exotoxin, which enters the enterocyte, that is the major cause of the secretory diarrhoea (**142b, 48**). *Escherichia coli* O157 shows the complexity of the pathogenic properties of the intestinal pathogens. It produces an adhesin necessary for attachment of the organism to the intestinal wall, a haemolysin, and verotoxin or shiga-like toxin.

Invasion of the mucosal layer of the colon is a characteristic of *Shigella* spp. (**143**). Here effacement of enterocytes occurs, cells are killed and the bacteria spread to neighbouring cells. With the inflammatory response, neutrophils accumulate, microabscesses form and local bleeding also occurs. A bloody stool containing pus can be a feature of shigella infection. Penetration through the mucosa and submucosa into lymphoid tissue is characteristic of *Salmonella typhi* (**144**). Diarrhoea is not common and enteric fever is characterized by fever and malaise. The organisms enter the blood and thus in suspected typhoid or enteric fever the collection of blood cultures is essential.

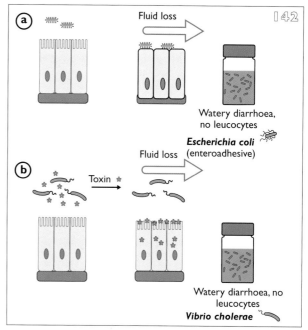

142 (a) Bacteria such as enteroadhesive *Escherichia coli* adhere to the surface of the enterocyte, causing effacement. **(b)** While also causing effacement, *Vibrio cholerae* produces an exotoxin that results in the secretory diarrhoea.

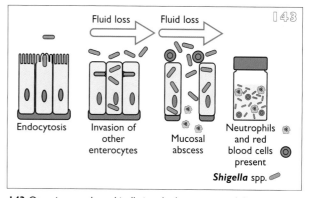

143 Organisms such as shigella invade the mucosa and destroy enterocytes; microabscess formation occurs. The stool contains blood and pus cells.

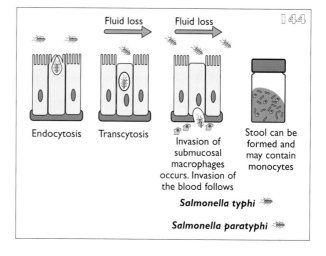

144 Salmonella penetrates the mucosa and submucosa.

Antibiotic-associated diarrhoea is an important entity in many hospitals and is a significant cause of morbidity in the older patient. *Clostridium difficile* is the main agent of the condition; the patient may have low numbers of organisms amongst their bowel flora on admission to hospital, or spores may be acquired from the hospital environment. Most antibiotics have an effect on the normal flora of the colon, and the imbalance that results allows *Clostridium difficile* to overgrow. Multiplying bacteria produce two proteins A and B, which (unlike the toxin of *Vibrio cholerae*) both act as toxins. The resulting diarrhoea may progress to pseudomembranous colitis (**145**).

Endogenous organisms

When a faecolith obstructs the lumen of the appendix, bacteria multiply behind the obstruction to produce appendicitis. This can progress to an abscess, rupture, and the development of peritonitis. Organisms can also travel via the portal vein to the liver and initiate a liver abscess (**146**).

In older patients diverticular disease of the descending colon is not uncommon. Here the mucosal and submucosal layers of the colon herniate through the muscle layer. Inflammation and the muscles of the colon itself may obstruct the opening of the diverticulum. Trapped bacteria multiply, with the resulting inflammation progressing to abscess formation. The same consequences of an appendix abscess may arise.

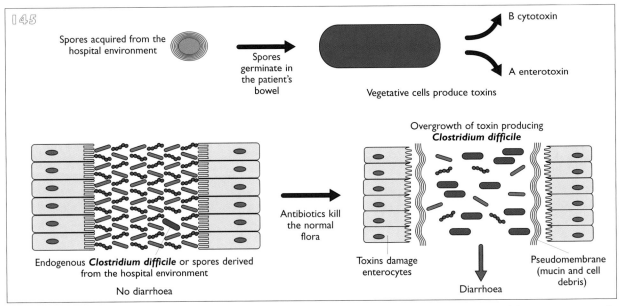

145 Spores of *Clostridium difficile* germinate to produce vegetative cells, which synthesize toxins A and B. Overgrowth of the organism can result in antibiotic-associated diarrhoea.

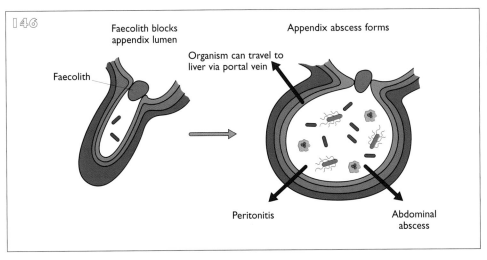

146 If the lumen of the appendix is obstructed by a faecolith, the trapped normal flora reproduce behind the obstruction.

Infections of the biliary tract can arise as a result of some pathology in its lumen, wall or outside. One example is the presence of a gallstone in the gall bladder itself or within the lumen of the common bile duct. It is reasonable to assume that there may be small numbers of bowel bacteria in the biliary tract. They only become relevant when normal function is compromised, for example by an impacted stone (**147a, b**). The bacteria proliferate behind the obstruction and biliary tract sepsis arises. In addition to local infection, bacteria can spread to the peritoneum and enter the blood to initiate sepsis.

Bacteria from the bowel can reach the liver by two routes, the biliary tract and the portal vein. Here again the common bacteria of the bowel are involved (**148**).

Peritonitis

Peritonitis can be divided into primary and secondary. In primary peritonitis there is no defined source. In the patient with liver cirrhosis, bacteria from the portal vein are not cleared by the macrophages of the liver. In the setting of portal hypertension, these bacteria may be shunted via the peri-hepatic lymphatics, from where they leak into the peritoneal space and initiate infection.

Secondary peritonitis arises from a defined source where there is compromise of the integrity of the bowel (**149**). Pelvic inflammatory disease (PID) in the female can also lead to secondary peritonitis as the Fallopian tubes open into the peritoneum.

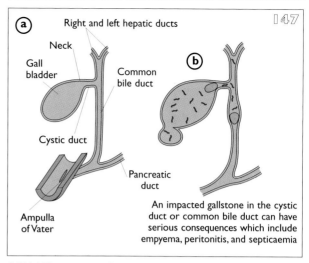

An impacted gallstone in the cystic duct or common bile duct can have serious consequences which include empyema, peritonitis, and septicaemia

147 (**a**) The structure of the hepatobiliary system. (**b**) Stones in the gall bladder or common bile duct lead to hepatobiliary sepsis.

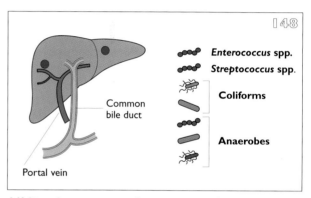

Enterococcus spp.
Streptococcus spp.
Coliforms
Anaerobes

148 Liver abscesses can arise from two sources. Consider these bacteria at least.

149 Compromise of the integrity of the bowel mucosa by a number of mechanisms can result in peritonitis. In the female patient, organisms from pelvic inflammatory disease must also be considered.

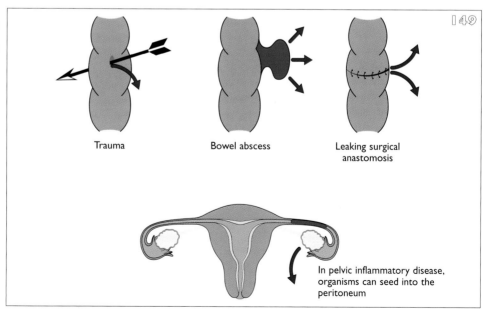

Trauma

Bowel abscess

Leaking surgical anastomosis

In pelvic inflammatory disease, organisms can seed into the peritoneum

Diagnosis

Pain typical of disease of the teeth and gums should bring the patient to the dentist. Dyspepsia and pain associated with duodenal ulcers should alert the clinician to *Helicobacter pylori* infection when other causes such as aspirin or non-steroidal anti-inflammatory drug (NSAID) use have been excluded. Disease caused by this organism can be identified or screened for by a number of tests (**150**). Clearly endoscopy, biopsy, and histopathological examination are the gold standards; culture may also be done here. The urease test relies on the fact that the potent urease produced by *Helicobacter pylori* converts ^{13}C urea to products which include $^{13}CO_2$. After swallowing labelled urea, any exhaled and labelled CO_2 can be measured. Antibody tests can be used to measure helicobacter IgG antibody levels.

Acute vomiting 1–6 hours after consuming food should alert the clinician to acute food poisoning by organisms producing emetic toxins, such as *Staphylococcus aureus* and *Bacillus cereus*. In any diarrhoeal illness a patient should be asked about recent food and travel history. It is important to record this information on the request form accompanying a specimen. Travel to underdeveloped parts of the world would widen the tests done, and would include, for example, testing the stool for *Vibrio cholerae*. In this setting the ova and cysts of parasites should also be looked for. Stool is plated on various solid media, which are then incubated in the atmospheric conditions needed to grow relevant bacteria. Selective enrichment media and further tests are also used to determine if the specimen contains one or more bacterial pathogens. An outline of the methods used to process a stool is shown in **151**. In countries such as the United Kingdom, stool specimens are routinely examined for the water-borne protozoal parasite cryptosporidium.

The diagnosis of infections of the small and large intestines, peritoneum, and hepatobiliary system must rely on clinical diagnosis first. For a bacteriological diagnosis, the specimen that must always be collected is blood for culture. If the patient has diarrhoea and an infective cause is likely, it is reasonable to send stool for culture. When pus is aspirated from an organ such as the liver or is found at laparotomy in the peritoneum, it should be sent as pus and not on a swab. Anaerobes survive much better in pus than on a swab!

In the hospitalized patient who has been prescribed antibiotics and who has diarrhoea, stool should be tested for the presence of *Clostridium difficile* and/or its toxins. Laboratories can use an EIA or tissue culture to test stool specimens for the presence of the toxins.

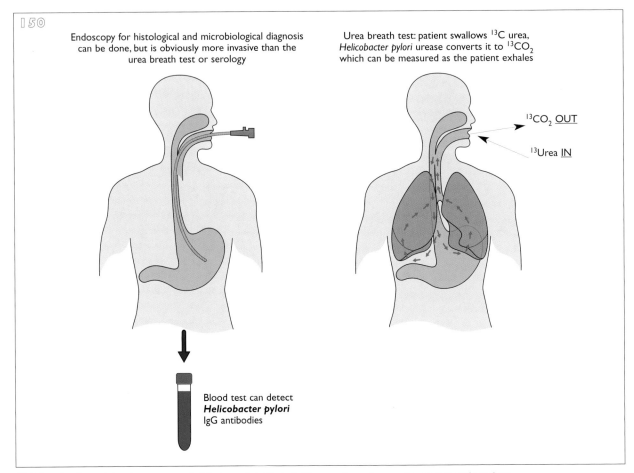

150

Endoscopy for histological and microbiological diagnosis can be done, but is obviously more invasive than the urea breath test or serology

Urea breath test: patient swallows ^{13}C urea, *Helicobacter pylori* urease converts it to $^{13}CO_2$ which can be measured as the patient exhales

$^{13}CO_2$ OUT

^{13}Urea IN

Blood test can detect **Helicobacter pylori** IgG antibodies

150 Tests for determining the presence of *Helicobacter pylori* include biopsy, culture, the urea breath test, and serology.

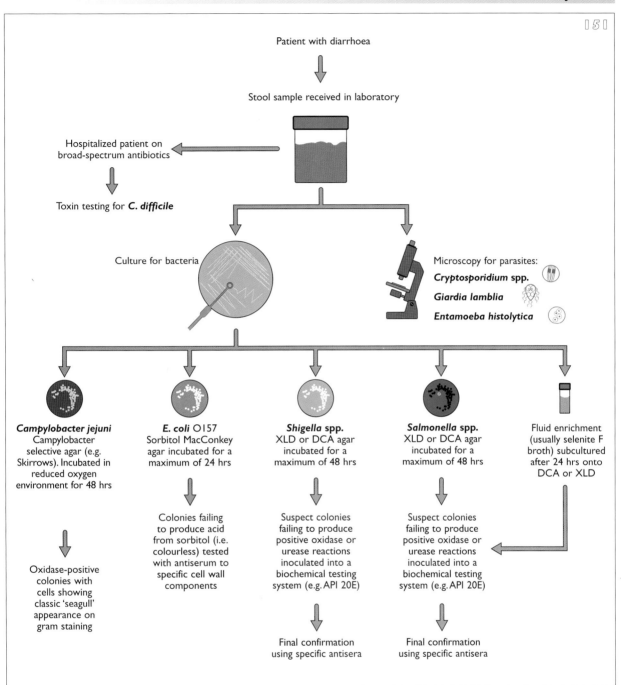

151 When a stool specimen is submitted to the laboratory, various procedures are conducted.

Treatment

An outline of treatment options is shown in **152**. Note that for exogenous organisms that cause gastroenteritis, supportive treatment with fluids and rest is usually sufficient. The patient with cholera may suffer massive fluid loss and intravenous fluids must be used to replace this loss. With *Escherichia coli* O157 the uncommon but severe end result of infection can be renal failure, requiring renal transplantation. Occasionally antibiotics such as ciprofloxacin may be used to shorten the duration of a bacterial diarrhoeal illness. However, antibiotics should not be used to treat *Escherichia coli* O157 infections, as they are considered to contribute to release of toxin from the bacterial cell, exacerbating the overall effect of the toxin.

In abdominal sepsis antibiotics that are active against streptococci, gram-negative coliforms, and anaerobes must be used. A cephalosporin such as cefuroxime with metronidazole is a reasonable first option. For broader cover, including enterococci, amoxycillin, gentamicin, and metronidazole is a useful combination. Another alternative is co-amoxiclav plus gentamicin. In the hospitalized patient where more resistant gram-negatives such as enterobacter and pseudomonas may be involved, piperacillin/tazobactam and gentamicin or a carbapenem and gentamicin can be appropriate. In the penicillin allergic patient with an immediate reaction to the β-lactam antibiotics, a combination of vancomycin, gentamicin or ciprofloxacin, and metronidazole could be considered. Clearly broad-spectrum antibiotic prescription must be modified when individual bacteria are isolated and identified. For example, if only anaerobes are isolated from pus and blood culture, metronidazole could be continued alone.

Public health issues

In general, the most important issue in the prevention of gastrointestinal illness is the quality of water and food that is consumed. Some of the preventive procedures that can be taken to reduce the incidence of disease are shown in **153**. These examples highlight that education and awareness, the supply of appropriate facilities and the

152

EXOGENOUS			ENDOGENOUS	
Organism	**Treatment**		**Organism**	**Treatment**
Campylobacter spp.	Supportive, occasionally erythromycin		*Streptococcus sanguis*	Dental care, amoxycillin, clindamycin as needed
Salmonella enteritidis	Supportive, occasionally ciprofloxacin		*Streptococcus mutans*	Dental care, amoxycillin, clindamycin as needed
Salmonella typhimurium	Supportive, occasionally ciprofloxacin		*Prevotella* spp.	Dental care, metronidazole, clindamycin as needed
Shigella dysenteriae	Supportive, occasionally ciprofloxacin		*Porphyromonas* spp.	Dental care, metronidazole, clindamycin as needed
Shigella flexneri	Supportive, occasionally ciprofloxacin		*Fusobacterium* spp.	Dental care, metronidazole, clindamycin as needed
Shigella boydii	Supportive, occasionally ciprofloxacin			
Shigella sonnei	Supportive		*Streptococcus* spp.	Amoxycillin, co-amoxiclav, cefuroxime, vancomycin
Escherichia coli O157	Supportive, dialysis, renal transplantation, NO antibiotics		*Enterococcus* spp.	Amoxycillin, co-amoxiclav, vancomycin
Salmonella typhi	Supportive, ciprofloxacin		Coliforms (e.g. *E. coli*)	Gentamicin, cefotaxime, ciprofloxacin, co-amoxiclav
Salmonella paratyphi	Supportive, ciprofloxacin		*Klebsiella* spp.	Gentamicin, ciprofloxacin, carbapenem
Vibrio cholerae	Supportive		*Bacteroides* spp.	Metronidazole, co-amoxiclav
Staphylococcus aureus	Supportive		*Peptostreptococcus/ Peptococcus* spp.	Metronidazole, co-amoxiclav
Bacillus cereus	Supportive		*Clostridium* spp.	Metronidazole, co-amoxiclav
Helicobacter pylori	Amoxycillin, clarithromycin, proton pump inhibitors			
Clostridium difficile	Metronidazole, vancomycin p.o.			

152 Some examples of the treatment options considered in infections of the alimentary canal. (p.o.: by mouth.)

correct storage of food are essential in preventing disease. In a developed country, the water supplied by utility companies is usually of the required quality for human consumption. However, on occasion organisms such as the protozoal parasite cryptosporidium occur in such numbers in storage dams or lakes that they cannot be removed by standard water purification procedures. The organisms thus enter the water supply and outbreaks of gastro-enteritis arise. This may happen when heavy rain washes large quantities of faecal matter from grazing farm animals into a storage dam supplying the purification plant.

Private water supplies may also be contaminated with animal effluent, and cryptosporidium and *Escherichia coli* O157 are organisms that can cause problems here. Contaminated water is the main source of epidemics of gastrointestinal infection in underdeveloped parts of the world and in refugee camps. This makes the supply of clean water one of the main concerns of aid agencies.

Despite improvement in regulations to improve food safety in developed parts of the world, outbreaks of diarrhoea and vomiting due to consumption of contaminated food are still reported. Bacteria such as *Salmonella enteriditis* are associated with raw eggs and can cause massive outbreaks. In 1994 for example, there was an outbreak of salmonella infection in the United States associated with a brand of ice cream, where the ingredients had been contaminated with raw egg material containing the organism. About 250,000 people were affected nationally. The food industry is an international business nowadays. Raspberries contaminated with a cyclosporan parasite caused an outbreak of gastrointestinal disease in the United States and Canada. This fresh fruit had been imported from Guatemala where it had been contaminated in the fields by bird faeces.

It is important that the international traveller who goes to either urban or rural areas is aware of the risks of water and food-borne disease. They should be advised to use either bottled water or boil fresh water. Food should be carefully selected and properly cooked. Fresh fruit and vegetables of dubious origin should be avoided. A wide range of organisms can cause 'travellers diarrhoea'. Some advocate the use of prophylactic antibiotic such as ciprofloxacin, which would be effective against an organism such as shigella. Certain gastrointestinal infections can be prevented by vaccination. Organisms for which vaccines are available include *Salmonella typhi* and *Vibrio cholerae*.

The essential responsibility of the medical doctor either in the community or in hospital is to ensure that any case of food poisoning is notified to the local public health department or CCDC. In the United Kingdom for example, there is a statutory responsibility to do this. Specimens should also be collected for referral to the laboratory. This is the only way that a potential outbreak can be identified and controlled, either in a family, school or wider community, and future episodes prevented.

Comment

The wide range of toxins produced by bacteria characterizes the pathogenesis of infections of the gastrointestinal tract. More details of these toxins can be found in any comprehensive text such as Mandell, Douglas, and Bennett's *Principles and Practice of Infectious Diseases*. The following review article is also an interesting article for further reading:

Royal RK, Hirano I (1996). The enteric nervous system. *New England Journal of Medicine* 334: 1106–14.

Public health aspects such as traveller's diarrhoea, and the epidemiological investigations of national and international food poisoning outbreaks are found in the following articles:

DuPont HL, Ericsson CD (1993). Prevention and treatment of traveller's diarrhoea. *New England Journal of Medicine* 328: 1821–6.
Hennessy TW, Hedberg CW, Slutsker L *et al.* (1996). A national outbreak of *Salmonella enteriditis* infections from ice cream. *New England Journal of Medicine* 334: 1821–6.
Herwaldt BL, Ackers M-L, The Cyclospora Working Group (1997). An outbreak of cyclosporiasis associated with imported raspberries. *New England Journal of Medicine* 336: 1548–56.

Source	Public health intervention
Campylobacter spp.	Maintenance of best practices in chicken farms. Store food at 3–5°C. Store raw food separately from cooked. Ensure (educate) that food is properly cooked
Escherichia coli O157	Educate farmers, teachers, and parents about the risks. Avoid direct contact with animals. Provide adequate hand washing facilities
Home-made mayonnaise made using raw eggs *Salmonella enteritidis*	Restrict the use of raw eggs in food. Store any food products containing raw egg at 3–5°C. Ensure that food is consumed promptly
Playschool *Shigella* spp.	Educate teachers, parents, and children about risks and the need for personal hygiene. Keep sick children away from school. Ensure adequate hand washing and toilet facilities
Nasal carriage in cook, contaminated food during preparation *Staphylococcus aureus*	Maintain best procedures in food preparation. Educate catering staff about risks. Store food at 3–5°C. Ensure adequate hand washing facilities

153 Some simple public health interventions that can be used to prevent community acquired gastrointestinal disease.

7 Infections of the Respiratory Tract

Introduction

The list of organisms that can cause disease in the respiratory tract is extensive and includes pneumococcus, haemophilus, group A streptococcus, *Mycoplasma pneumoniae*, *Chlamydia pneumoniae*, and *Mycobacterium tuberculosis*. Important viruses to consider are influenza, parainfluenza, respiratory syncytial virus (RSV), and the 'common cold' rhinoviruses. In countries where vaccination programs are in place, diphtheria, whooping cough, and epiglottitis caused by *Haemophilus influenzae* b are uncommon. Where vaccination programs are poor these agents remain important as evidenced for example by the increase in diphtheria in parts of Eastern Europe in the 1990s.

Most of the organisms considered in this chapter have a human source, and it is reasonable to assume that they circulate within communities by spread from an infected individual to susceptible individuals. Certain organisms such as influenza virus are known to spread nationally and internationally as epidemics or pandemics. Recognized pathogens such as pneumococcus also exist in individuals as part of the normal flora of the upper respiratory tract. *Mycobacterium tuberculosis*, which has infected about one third of the world's population, would never be regarded as part of the normal flora.

Other pathogens can be acquired from animals; these infections are termed zoonoses. Examples are Q fever associated with farm animals, which is caused by *Coxiella burnetii*, and psittacosis associated with birds such as parrots, which is caused by *Chlamydia psittaci*. Water is the source of *Legionella pneumophila*, the cause of Legionnaires' disease. This bacterium can survive in water over a wide range of temperatures, and grows in water where the temperature is between 25°C and 45°C. Any water supply in this temperature range may contain the organism in significant numbers. If this water is aerosolized as a fine mist, inhalation of these droplets may give rise to legionellosis. Ubiquitous fungi such as aspergillus and *Pneumocystis carinii* are important pathogens of the respiratory tract in the immunocompromised patient. Some examples of the sources of infections are shown in **154a–d**.

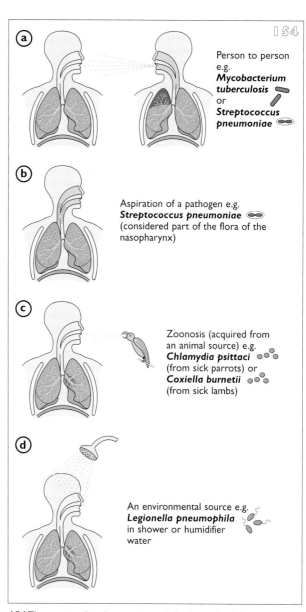

154 The routes whereby respiratory infections arise: (**a**) person to person; (**b**) aspiration; (**c**) acquired from an animal source, e.g. psittacosis; (**d**) acquired from an environmental source.

Anatomically, the respiratory system can be divided into the upper and lower tracts. The upper tract consists of the middle ear, mastoid cavity, nasal sinuses, and nasopharynx, while the lower tract extends from the larynx to the lungs. All these structures can be involved in infection, and while certain organisms such as legionella are restricted to one anatomical site, the lungs, others such as pneumococcus can cause middle ear infection, sinusitis and pneumonia. Some important defences of the respiratory tract, based on normal anatomy, physiology and immune function are outlined in **155a**. Compromise of these defences predisposes to infection (**155b**).

Pneumonia is a disease of the lung parenchyma, which can be divided into community acquired pneumonia (CAP) and hospital acquired pneumonia (HAP). These terms are useful as different organisms can be considered in the community and hospital settings. HAP is that which arises 48 hours after admission of the patient to hospital. While some of the agents that cause CAP may be involved, HAP is usually associated with 'coliforms', *Pseudomonas aeruginosa*, and *Staphylococcus aureus* including MRSA.

In the community, typical lobar pneumonia is characterized by fever, chest pain, and production of purulent sputum, whereas atypical pneumonia is characterized by dyspnoea and a cough, with minimal sputum production. Organisms associated with atypical pneumonia include *Mycoplasma pneumoniae*, *Chlamydia pneumoniae*, *Chlamydia psittaci*, *Coxiella burnetii*, and *Legionella pneumophila*.

Lung abscess may arise as a complication of certain bacterial pneumonias, following aspiration of oral bacteria, from septic emboli arising from right-sided endocarditis, or from thrombophlebitis of the great veins of the neck or the pelvis. Abscesses may also arise distal to an obstruction in the bronchial tree, such as a carcinoma.

The microbiology of the lung in the cystic fibrosis patient is also considered. The abnormal physiology of the lung in these individuals provides a site for chronic infection by certain bacteria, which contributes significantly to the morbidity and mortality of this condition.

Organisms

A list of important bacteria that cause infection of the respiratory tract is shown in **156**. These have been grouped according to the anatomical sites of the respiratory system where they can cause disease.

In the cystic fibrosis patient *Staphylococcus aureus*, *Haemophilus influenzae*, *Pseudomonas aeruginosa*, and *Burkholderia cepacia* are important. While the first three agents are recognized human pathogens, the latter organism is of plant origin, and reflects the unique environment of the cystic fibrosis lung that enables this organism to grow here. Because of its resistance to many common antibiotics, burkholderia is particularly challenging to treat. Other organisms such as atypical mycobacteria may also be of relevance in the patient with cystic fibrosis.

Some features of organisms associated with atypical pneumonia are shown in **157**. Legionella is an intracellular pathogen. It is phagocytosed by alveolar macrophages, but is able to escape the killing mechanism of the phagolysosome.

Following multiplication, the macrophage ruptures and the released bacteria infect other cells. Mycoplasmas are free-living bacteria that lack a cell wall. *Mycoplasma pneumoniae* probably attaches to the respiratory epithelium by a terminal P1 protein structure. This organism can cause pharyngitis, tracheitis, bronchitis and pneumonia.

Chlamydia are a unique class of bacteria that are obligate intracellular parasites. *Coxiella burnetii*, the causative agent of Q fever, is a member of the Rickettsiaceae, which are also obligate intracellular parasites. *Coxiella burnetii* is unusual as it is able to survive desiccation and can be wind-borne. Outbreaks of Q fever have been recorded downwind of farms where there were infected animals.

Pathogenesis
Otitis media, mastoiditis and sinusitis

The middle ear, mastoid cavity and sinuses are connected either directly or indirectly to the nasopharynx. The ciliated respiratory epithelium, which lines the sinuses and Eustachian tube, pushes mucus out of these structures and any trapped bacteria are removed. In middle ear and sinus infection it is likely that viruses such as RSV invade this epithelium, destroy the cells and compromise the mucociliary function allowing bacteria to enter sterile areas (**158a**). Although mastoid disease is uncommon, it is important to recognize this condition. Bacteria can spread from the middle ear to the mastoid cavity via the aditus. Because of the proximity of the mastoid cavity to the middle cranial fossa, lateral venous sinus and jugular bulb, mastoiditis can have serious complications (**158b, c**).

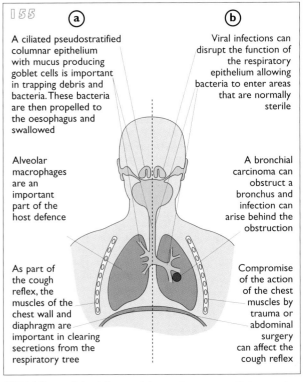

155 (**a**) Some of the defences of the respiratory tract that prevent infection. (**b**) Compromise of these defences increases the likelihood of infection.

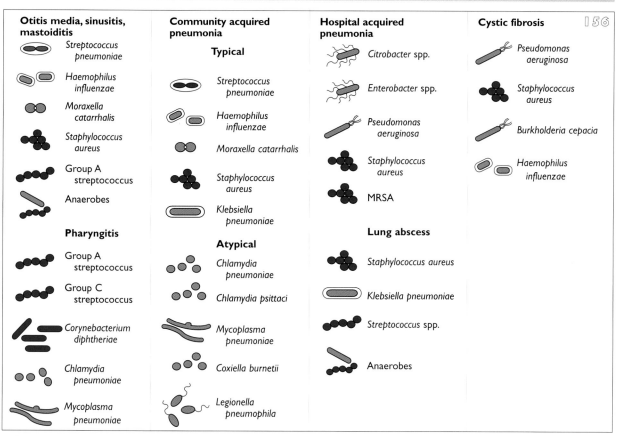

Otitis media, sinusitis, mastoiditis

- *Streptococcus pneumoniae*
- *Haemophilus influenzae*
- *Moraxella catarrhalis*
- *Staphylococcus aureus*
- Group A streptococcus
- Anaerobes

Pharyngitis

- Group A streptococcus
- Group C streptococcus
- *Corynebacterium diphtheriae*
- *Chlamydia pneumoniae*
- *Mycoplasma pneumoniae*

Community acquired pneumonia

Typical

- *Streptococcus pneumoniae*
- *Haemophilus influenzae*
- *Moraxella catarrhalis*
- *Staphylococcus aureus*
- *Klebsiella pneumoniae*

Atypical

- *Chlamydia pneumoniae*
- *Chlamydia psittaci*
- *Mycoplasma pneumoniae*
- *Coxiella burnetii*
- *Legionella pneumophila*

Hospital acquired pneumonia

- *Citrobacter* spp.
- *Enterobacter* spp.
- *Pseudomonas aeruginosa*
- *Staphylococcus aureus*
- MRSA

Lung abscess

- *Staphylococcus aureus*
- *Klebsiella pneumoniae*
- *Streptococcus* spp.
- Anaerobes

Cystic fibrosis

- *Pseudomonas aeruginosa*
- *Staphylococcus aureus*
- *Burkholderia cepacia*
- *Haemophilus influenzae*

156 A list of organisms that can cause disease in the respiratory tract. (MRSA: methicillin resistant *Staphylococcus aureus*.)

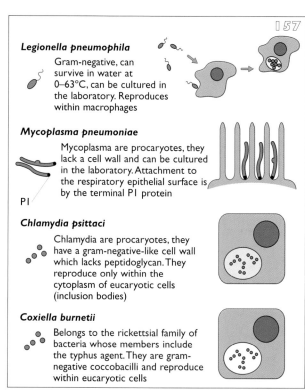

Legionella pneumophila

Gram-negative, can survive in water at 0–63°C, can be cultured in the laboratory. Reproduces within macrophages

Mycoplasma pneumoniae

Mycoplasma are procaryotes, they lack a cell wall and can be cultured in the laboratory. Attachment to the respiratory epithelial surface is by the terminal P1 protein

P1

Chlamydia psittaci

Chlamydia are procaryotes, they have a gram-negative-like cell wall which lacks peptidoglycan. They reproduce only within the cytoplasm of eucaryotic cells (inclusion bodies)

Coxiella burnetii

Belongs to the rickettsial family of bacteria whose members include the typhus agent. They are gram-negative coccobacilli and reproduce within eucaryotic cells

157 Some features of certain organisms associated with 'atypical' pneumonia.

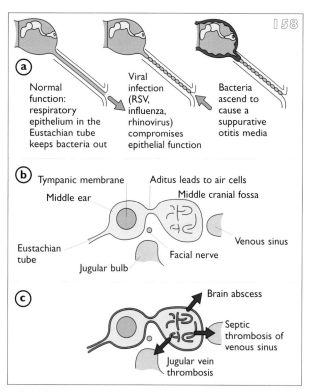

(a)

Normal function: respiratory epithelium in the Eustachian tube keeps bacteria out

Viral infection (RSV, influenza, rhinovirus) compromises epithelial function

Bacteria ascend to cause a suppurative otitis media

(b) Tympanic membrane — Aditus leads to air cells

Middle ear — Middle cranial fossa

Eustachian tube — Venous sinus

Jugular bulb — Facial nerve

(c) Brain abscess

Septic thrombosis of venous sinus

Jugular vein thrombosis

158 (a) Compromise of the respiratory epithelium in the Eustachian tube allows bacteria to enter the middle ear. (b) The relationship of the mastoid air cells to other structures. (c) Infection in the mastoid cavity can spread to neighbouring structures.

Pharyngitis

A range of bacteria can cause pharyngitis (**156**); viruses such as influenza, adenovirus, HSV, and Epstein Barr virus (EBV) should also be considered. Group A streptococcus, *Streptococcus pyogenes,* is the classic cause of pharyngitis or 'strep throat'. One of the major virulence factors of this organism is the surface M protein, which has antiphagocytic properties. In addition, secreted extracellular proteins such as the haemolysins O and S, DNase, NADase, streptokinase, and the pyrogenic toxin account in part for the range of diseases that this organism can cause in addition to pharyngitis (**159**). These include scarlet fever, TSS, and cellulitis.

Group A streptococcus may precipitate peritonsillar abscess or quinsy, but anaerobes should always be considered as well. A complication of the condition is septic thrombophlebitis of the jugular vein.

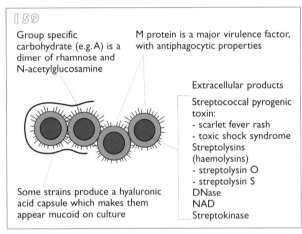

159

Group specific carbohydrate (e.g. A) is a dimer of rhamnose and N-acetylglucosamine

M protein is a major virulence factor, with antiphagocytic properties

Extracellular products

Streptococcal pyrogenic toxin:
- scarlet fever rash
- toxic shock syndrome
Streptolysins (haemolysins)
- streptolysin O
- streptolysin S
DNase
NAD
Streptokinase

Some strains produce a hyaluronic acid capsule which makes them appear mucoid on culture

159 Some of the pathogenic properties of group A streptococcus, many of which are involved in the development of 'strep throat'.

Pneumonia

Pneumonia usually arises as a result of aspiration of a pathogen such as pneumococcus into the lung in such numbers that they overwhelm the local defences. The establishment of pneumococcus infection depends on several factors. These include the number of organisms aspirated and the ability of the ciliated respiratory epithelium to remove these bacteria. The smoker, and the individual with COAD or heart failure is at risk.

Bacteria reproducing in the alveoli stimulate the local macrophages and an immune response is initiated. Classic pneumococcal lobar pneumonia is divided into four stages. These are the acute congestion stage, characterized by engorgement of the capillaries and recruitment of neutrophils into the lung parenchyma, then red hepatization where there is flow of RBCs from the capillaries into the alveolar space. The next stage is grey hepatization with large numbers of dead and dying neutrophils and degenerating RBCs. The last stage, resolution, starts with the arrival of specific antibodies.

By the very nature of the hospital environment where antibiotic use is significant, resistant bacteria are often present. These include enterobacter, citrobacter, *Pseudomonas aeruginosa,* and MRSA. It is reasonable to assume that the hospitalized patient is stressed, and one result of this is increased proteolytic activity in the saliva, which contributes to rapid turnover of the fibronectin layer that covers the epithelium of the pharynx. Fibronectin is considered to have the resident normal flora attached. Loss of fibronectin means that the attached normal flora is also lost. The exposed epithelium is then colonized by large numbers of gram-negative bacteria such as pseudomonas, which can be aspirated into the lungs (**160a**). Some of the other contributory factors in HAP are shown in **160b**.

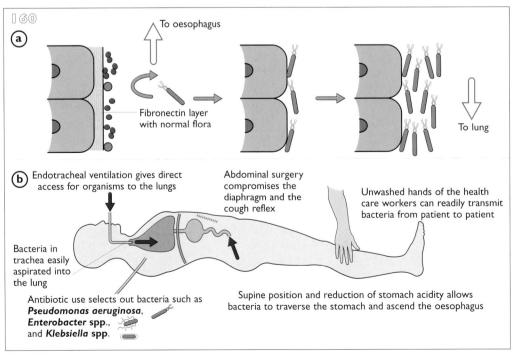

160

(a) To oesophagus

Fibronectin layer with normal flora

To lung

(b) Endotracheal ventilation gives direct access for organisms to the lungs

Abdominal surgery compromises the diaphragm and the cough reflex

Unwashed hands of the health care workers can readily transmit bacteria from patient to patient

Bacteria in trachea easily aspirated into the lung

Antibiotic use selects out bacteria such as **Pseudomonas aeruginosa**, **Enterobacter spp.**, and **Klebsiella spp.**

Supine position and reduction of stomach acidity allows bacteria to traverse the stomach and ascend the oesophagus

160 (a) Mucosal surfaces such as the oropharynx are coated with fibronectin and the normal flora. Removal of this protective layer allows gram-negative bacteria to colonize the oropharynx in significant numbers. (b) Some of the contributing factors to hospital aquired pneumonia.

Lung abscess

A lung abscess can arise as a complication of pneumonia, aspiration, or septic emboli (**161a, b**). With pneumonia caused by *Staphylococcus aureus* and *Klebsiella pneumoniae*, the inflammatory response can progress to local tissue necrosis and abscess formation. An abscess may also arise following the aspiration of fluid containing stomach contents and the bacteria of the oral cavity. This may occur in an obtunded or unconscious person and alcohol and epilepsy are relevant here. Any condition that compromises the swallowing function of the oesophagus or the anatomy of the trachea and bronchi can predispose to abscess formation. A lung abscess may arise as a result of compression of a bronchus and this may be the first indication of a bronchial carcinoma (**161c**). Septic emboli arising from thrombophlebitis of the veins of the neck or pelvis can lodge in the lung and progress to abscess formation. In the setting of tricuspid valve endocarditis, an embolus from a valve vegetation can also progress to an abscess.

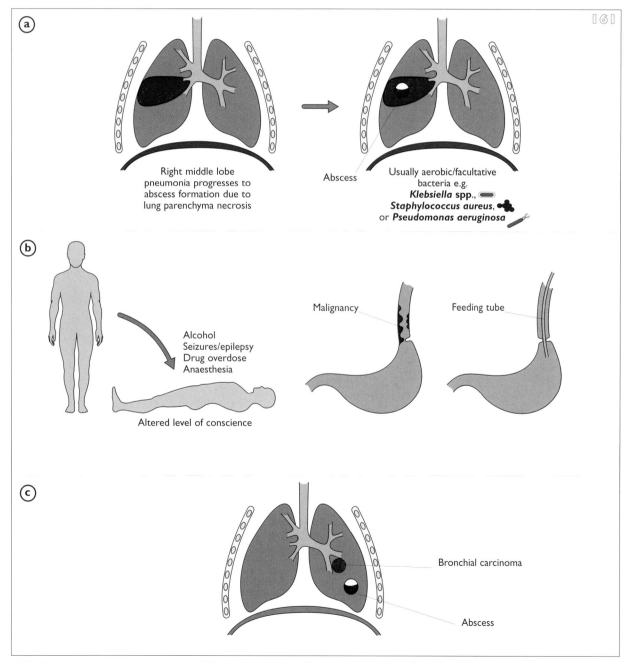

161 A lung abscess may arise as a result of: (**a**) bacterial pneumonia; (**b**) aspiration of stomach fluid and oral bacteria; (**c**) compression of a bronchus by a carcinoma.

Cystic fibrosis

Cystic fibrosis arises as a result of a defect in the cystic fibrosis transmembrane regulator (CFTR) protein coded by the CFTR gene. This defect affects a number of organ systems and production of viscous secretions alters normal function. It is in the lung that the condition is particularly relevant, as all adolescents and adults with cystic fibrosis have chronic suppurative lung disease. In early childhood, the lung becomes colonized with pseudomonas, which produces large amounts of extracellular mucoid alginate. *Staphylococcus aureus* and *Burkholderia cepacia* are two other organisms that can also colonize the lung. A vigorous inflammatory response, bacterial toxins and the products of dead neutrophils, in particular their viscous DNA, all contribute to the formation of the thick secretions that compromise lung function (**162a, b**). In adolescents and young adults the appearance of burkholderia in the respiratory secretions can be associated with rapid deterioration. For this reason patients whose sputum is positive for *Burkholderia cepacia* should be segregated from those whose sputum is free of the organism, in order to reduce the chance of spread.

Diagnosis

An outline of the microbiology tests that can be used to diagnose respiratory tract infection is shown in **163**. In most cases the diagnosis of otitis media or sinusitis, either as an acute or chronic infection, is made on clinical grounds and antibiotics may be prescribed. Radiography can be used in the diagnosis of sinusitis. On occasion an aspirate may be collected to identify the organisms present. With pharyngitis, a throat swab can be collected. Serological tests may also be done when the differential diagnosis includes mycoplasma and viruses such as EBV.

Pneumonia, either CAP, HAP or atypical, will initially be diagnosed clinically and by chest X-ray. For the microbiological diagnosis of infections of the lower respiratory tract, analysis of sputum is important. The isolation and identification of bacteria and determination of their antibiotic susceptibility are part of patient management. Blood cultures should be collected in suspected bacterial pneumonia.

The diagnosis of pulmonary TB may be straightforward when a patient with the symptoms and signs of the disease has TB confirmed promptly by a positive Ziehl-Neelsen (ZN) stain of the sputum. The diagnosis is usually not so obvious and it is always important to ask the question 'does this patient have TB?'

In the patient with an atypical pneumonia, identification of the causative agent can be more difficult, as these organisms are not routinely cultured in laboratories. A careful history, documenting exposure to birds, farm animals, or possible exposure to legionella, needs to be taken. Serological tests such as CFT are used in the identification of mycoplasma, psittacosis and Q fever. A four-fold or more increase in the titre, for example from 1/16 in an 'acute' serum taken at admission to 1/256 in a 'convalescent' serum taken 10–14 days later, would be considered diagnostic. The problem with the CFT is that it relies on two sera and thus takes 10 days or more for a result after the acute

presentation. A useful test in the setting of legionella infection is the urine antigen test, which can detect antigen to serogroup 1, the most common serogroup encountered.

On occasion the collection of sputum may not be possible. The patient may not be producing sputum or may be too ill. In these cases samples may be obtained by invasive procedures (**164a–c**). Endotracheal tube (ETT) aspirates are often collected from the ICU patient. It is important to appreciate that any organism isolated here may be colonizing the tube and not be relevant to the actual infection in the lung. For this reason more invasive procedures such as a bronchial lavage or brush specimen may be used. Where present, pleural effusions should be aspirated and a pleural biopsy considered.

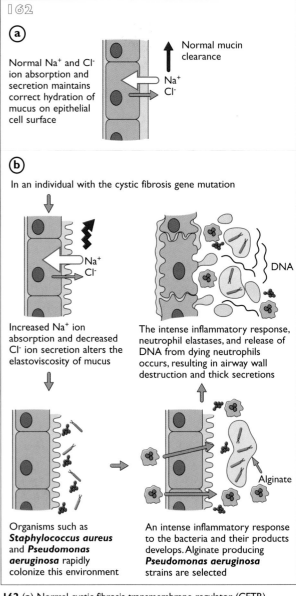

162 (a) Normal cystic fibrosis transmembrane regulator (CFTR) protein function. **(b)** In cystic fibrosis patients the malfunctioning of the CFTR protein produces an environment that is colonized by bacteria.

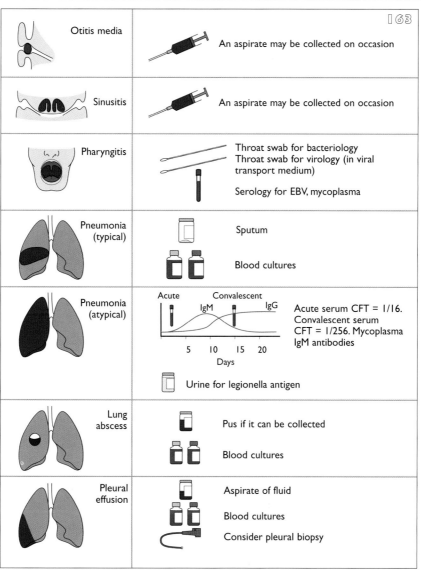

163 Tests to consider in the diagnosis of respiratory tract infection. (CFT: complement fixation test; EBV: Epstein Barr virus; Ig: immunoglobulin.)

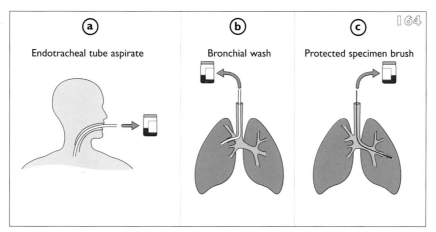

164 With the ICU patient, various invasive diagnostic procedures can be used to obtain a specimen: (**a**) endotracheal tube aspirate; (**b**) bronchial lavage; (**c**) protected specimen brush.

Examination of sputum from the cystic fibrosis patient requires the use of selective media to isolate *Staphylococcus aureus* and *Burkholderia cepacia*, as mucoid *Pseudomonas aeruginosa* overwhelms other bacteria on standard blood agar plates (**165**). A chocolate blood agar plate incubated anaerobically is useful to select for haemophilus, as pseudomonas will not grow under anaerobic conditions.

Treatment

Antibiotics to consider in infection of the respiratory tract are shown in **166**. For the treatment of otitis media and sinusitis supportive treatment with decongestants is often appropriate, but antibiotics such as amoxycillin may be given on occasion. Group A streptococcal pharyngitis can be treated with oral penicillin V.

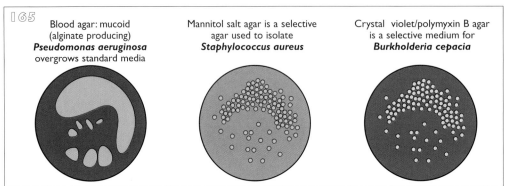

165 Blood agar: mucoid (alginate producing) ***Pseudomonas aeruginosa*** overgrows standard media

Mannitol salt agar is a selective agar used to isolate ***Staphylococcus aureus***

Crystal violet/polymyxin B agar is a selective medium for ***Burkholderia cepacia***

165 In sputum specimens from cystic fibrosis patients, *Pseudomonas aeruginosa* overwhelms other bacteria. Selective media are used to isolate *Staphylococcus aureus* and *Burkholderia cepacia*.

166

Otitis media, sinusitis, mastoiditis

Streptococcus pneumoniae	Amoxycillin, erythromycin
Haemophilus influenzae	Amoxycillin, ciprofloxacin
Moraxella catarrhalis	Co-amoxiclav, clarithromycin, ciprofloxacin
Staphylococcus aureus	Flucloxacillin, erythromycin, ciprofloxacin
Group A streptococcus	Amoxycillin, benzylpenicillin
Anaerobes	Metronidazole, co-amoxiclav

Pharyngitis

Group A streptococcus	Benzylpenicillin, amoxycillin
Group C streptococcus	Benzylpenicillin, amoxycillin
Corynebacterium diphtheriae	Benzylpenicillin, erythromycin (antitoxin)
Chlamydia pneumoniae	Erythromycin, tetracycline
Mycoplasma pneumoniae	Erythromycin, tetracycline

Community acquired pneumonia

Typical

Streptococcus pneumoniae	Amoxycillin, erythromycin, cefuroxime
Haemophilus influenzae	Amoxycillin, cefuroxime, ciprofloxacin
Moraxella catarrhalis	Co-amoxiclav, cefuroxime, ciprofloxacin
Staphylococcus aureus	Flucloxacillin, erythromycin
Klebsiella pneumoniae	Cefuroxime, gentamicin

Atypical

Chlamydia pneumoniae	Erythromycin, tetracycline
Chlamydia psittaci	Erythromycin, tetracycline
Mycoplasma pneumoniae	Erythromycin
Coxiella burnetii	Erythromycin, tetracycline
Legionella pneumophila	Erythromycin (and rifampicin)

Hospital acquired pneumonia

Citrobacter spp.	Gentamicin, ciprofloxacin, imipenem
Enterobacter spp.	Gentamicin, ciprofloxacin, imipenem
Pseudomonas aeruginosa	Gentamicin, ciprofloxacin, imipenem
Staphylococcus aureus	Flucloxacillin (and gentamicin)
MRSA	Vancomycin (and gentamicin)

Lung abscess

Staphylococcus aureus	Flucloxacillin and gentamicin
Klebsiella pneumoniae	Cefuroxime and gentamicin
Streptococcus spp.	Benzylpenicillin, clindamycin
Anaerobes	Metronidazole, clindamycin

Cystic fibrosis

Pseudomonas aeruginosa	Gentamicin, ciprofloxacin, imipenem
Staphylococcus aureus	Flucloxacillin, gentamicin, imipenem
Burkholderia cepacia	Ciprofloxacin, ceftazidime, imipenem
Haemophilus influenzae	Ciprofloxacin, imipenem

166 Examples of appropriate antibiotics that may be used to treat certain respiratory conditions.

In pneumonia, the need for intravenous antibiotics is determined by the clinical assessment of the patient and factors such as heart rate (>120/minute), respiratory rate (>30/minute), and pyrexia (>39°C) are indications for giving intravenous antibiotics. Cefuroxime and erythromycin is one combination. Cefuroxime is effective against penicillin sensitive pneumococcus and is also resistant to the β-lactamase enzyme of moraxella and haemophilus. Erythromycin or clarithromycin is included when an agent that can cause an atypical pneumonia is likely. When the patient improves, intravenous antibiotics can be changed to oral agents. Some treatment regimes that may be considered for a number of community acquired conditions are shown in **167a, b**.

Hospital-acquired pneumonia

Here it is always prudent to consider *Pseudomonas aeruginosa*, citrobacter, enterobacter, and MRSA. An aminoglycoside such as gentamicin should be given by the pulse dose method in combination with a β-lactam such as co-amoxiclav. Piperacillin/tazobactam or the carbapenems imipenem or meropenem should usually be reserved for the ICU patient.

Lung abscess

Where there is a lung abscess caused by a specific organism, the antibiotic regime should be specific for that organism. In the case of a lung abscess arising as a result of aspiration of oral bacteria, agents effective against streptococci and anaerobes must be used. Metronidazole and penicillin is one combination; co-amoxiclav and clindamycin are alternatives. Antibiotics may need to be given for several months.

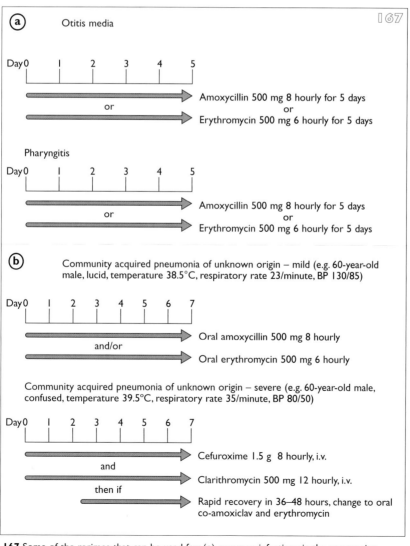

167 Some of the regimes that can be used for: **(a)** common infections in the community; **(b)** the treatment of community aquired pneumonia in the hospitalized patient.

Cystic fibrosis

An outline of the treatment for the cystic fibrosis patient is shown in **168**. For *Pseudomonas aeruginosa* agents such as ceftazidime, gentamicin, and imipenem are useful. If *Staphylococcus aureus* is present, flucloxacillin may be added; however, imipenem and gentamicin are also effective. *Burkholderia cepacia* is resistant to aminoglycosides and agents such as ceftazidime, imipenem, ciprofloxacin, and co-trimoxazole may be used.

Public health issues

Vaccination is of major importance in the prevention of infections of the respiratory tract. Vaccines include those for influenza, *Haemophilus influenzae* b, pneumococcus, diphtheria, and pertussis. These are examples of how modern science has contributed to reducing the morbidity and mortality associated with respiratory disease in parts of the world where vaccination is practised.

An important aspect of public health is the consideration and control of legionella in any water system where droplets may be aerosolized. This includes hot water supplies, air conditioning systems, and mist devices in hotels, hospitals, and indoor and outdoor displays. Good and bad practice in the design of a hot water supply in a hotel are shown in **169a, b**. When water is stored between 20°C and 45°C, legionella will grow. The poor hot water system (**169a**) consists of a tank that cannot be cleaned properly and sludge accumulates at the bottom, ideal for the growth of legionella.

When the demand for water is low, water entering the distribution is at the correct temperature of 60°C and is free of significant numbers of legionella. At peak times however, for example in the summer holidays, the high demand for water means that the water is not adequately heated, organisms from the sludge enter the hot water distributed to showers and guests may be at risk of the disease. In the good system (**169b**), a base drain means that sludge can be regularly cleaned out. A circulation pump and a second lower heating coil mean that even at peak time, hot water is distributed at 60°C, providing safe water at all times.

Comment

The following two articles are examples of the investigation of outbreaks of pneumococcal disease in the community. Investigations included molecular typing methods, and are thus useful examples of how outbreaks are managed:

Hoge CW, Reichler MR, Dominguez EA *et al.* (1994). An epidemic of pneumococcal disease in an overcrowded, inadequately ventilated jail. *New England Journal of Medicine* **331**: 643–7.

Nuorti JP, Butler JC, Crutcher JM *et al.* (1998). An outbreak of multidrug-resistant pneumococcal pneumonia and bacteraemia among unvaccinated nursing home residents. *New England Journal of Medicine* **338**: 1861–8.

Guidelines of the British Thoracic Society for the management of CAP in adults and children and the control and prevention of tuberculosis in the United Kingdom can be found at:

http://www.brit-thoracic.org.uk/guide/guidelines.html

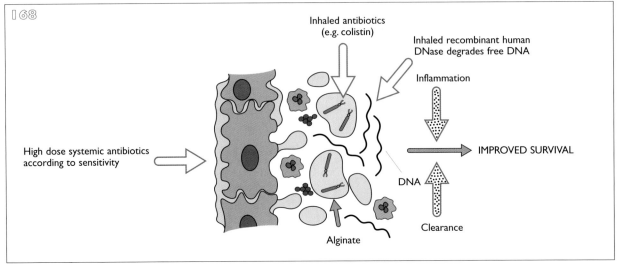

168 In addition to antibiotics, human DNase is also used in treatment of the cystic fibrosis patient.

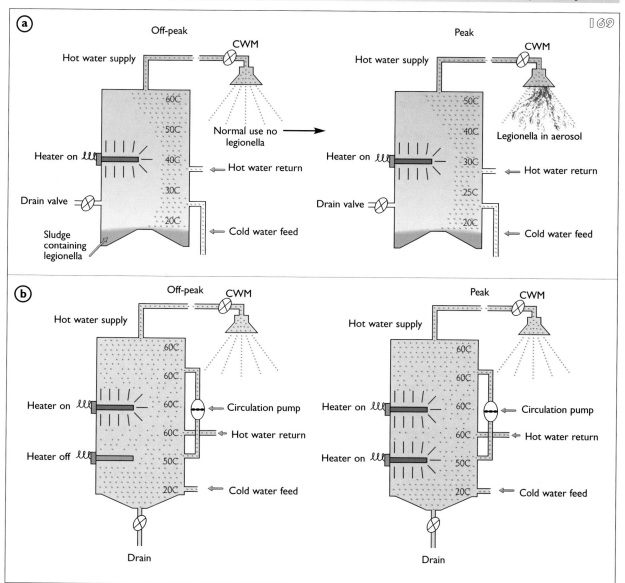

169 (a) A poor hot water supply system and **(b)** a good hot water system at 'off peak' and 'peak' times. (CWM: cold water mixer).

8 Tuberculosis

Introduction

It is estimated that over 1.7 billion people, or one-third of the world's population, are infected with *Mycobacterium tuberculosis* and that 3 million die each year from the disease. TB is thus responsible for more deaths than any other infectious agent. In countries such as the United Kingdom, the overall annual rate of the disease is about 10 cases/100,000, while in Africa this rate is in excess of 200 cases/100,000. A breakdown of the incidence in different ethnic groups in the United Kingdom reflects the rate in the countries of origin. For ethnic minorities who are classified as Black African, Indian subcontinent and Caribbean, the rates per 100,000 are >200, >100 and 20–30 respectively.

With the advent of effective anti-TB therapy in the 1950s, the control of the disease seemed a possibility. By the end of the twentieth century the situation had changed for the worse. The HIV epidemic is one important reason for this, as it increased the efficiency of the cycle of transmission. In sub-Saharan Africa it is estimated that about half of all the people with HIV are infected with *Mycobacterium tuberculosis*, and thus TB is the main AIDS defining illness. In addition, social problems of poverty and urban crowding exacerbate the issue and explain the high rates of disease in certain parts of the world.

Another issue is drug resistance. Treatment is prolonged, lasting for at least 6 months. If the services to supply and monitor treatment in each patient are under resourced, compliance can become a major issue. Non-compliance can result in the selection of mycobacteria that are resistant to one or more agents. Outbreaks of multi-drug resistant tuberculosis (MDR-TB) have occurred in hospitals, prisons and the community.

TB is a disease that has complex medical and social aspects, not just for one individual, but also for family, work, hospital, and social contacts. Prompt identification of the person with active lung disease is essential if spread of the organism to other individuals is to be limited. In the patient with a chronic cough, weight loss, and fever, and whose chest X-ray is characteristic of TB, the clinical diagnosis is usually obvious. A positive microscopy result will confirm the diagnosis. Unfortunately, patients are still admitted to hospital for other reasons, and the diagnosis of pulmonary TB is made days later when a chronic cough is noted or a chest X-ray is belatedly reviewed. As TB can arise in any organ, it is essential to ask the question 'does this patient have TB?' in the setting of weight loss and fever.

Organisms

A number of important bacteria belong to the genus *Mycobacterium*, and a classification of these organisms with some of the diseases they cause is shown in **170**. *Mycobacterium tuberculosis*, as with all other mycobacteria, is an obligate aerobic, rod shaped, non-spore forming organism. It is neither gram-positive nor gram-negative. Mycobacteria are 'acid-fast' and stain a deep magenta colour with ZN stain, for this reason they are referred to as acid-fast bacilli (AFB). The procedure for ZN staining is outlined in **171**. The acid-fast nature is due to the structure of the cell wall, whose constituents include complex lipids and mycolic acids. The heating process used in staining forces the carbol fuchsin into the cell, and it is the lipid barrier and complexing of the dye with the mycolic acid that prevents the organism from being decoloured by the acid alcohol. A photomicrograph of *Mycobacterium tuberculosis* in a sputum specimen stained by the ZN method is shown in **172**.

An outline of the cell wall structure of *Mycobacterium tuberculosis* is shown in **173**. Constituents of the cell wall are responsible for the pathogenic features of disease caused by *Mycobacterium tuberculosis*, characterized by overstimulation of the cell-mediated immune system.

170		
M. tuberculosis, M. bovis	Non-pigmented colonies	
M. kansasii	**Photochromogens** Pigmented colonies only when grown in light	Can cause disease in the damaged lung (e.g. COAD)
M. marinum		Can cause infections of the hand; acquired from tropical fish tanks
M. gordonae, M. xenopi	**Scotochromogens** Pigmented colonies when grown in light and dark	Can cause progressive lung disease
M. avium, M. intracellulare	**Non-pigmented colonies**	Can cause disseminated disease in AIDS patients
M. malmoense		Can cause progressive lung disease

170 A classification of mycobacteria that can cause disease in humans. Those not in the 'tuberculosis' group are classified according to growth characteristics. (AIDS: acquired immunodeficiency syndrome; COAD: chronic obstructive airways disease.)

171 The Ziehl-Neelsen stain. Carbol fuchsin enters the organism in the heating process. The subsequent decolourization step is unable to remove the stain.

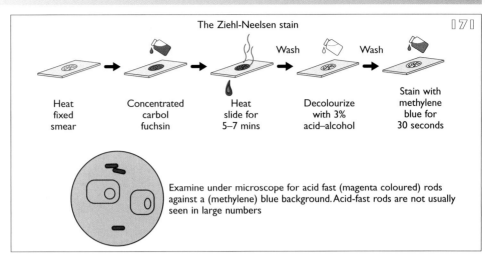

172 A photomicrograph of a sputum specimen stained by the Ziehl-Neelsen method. Numerous acid-fast bacilli are seen against the blue background.

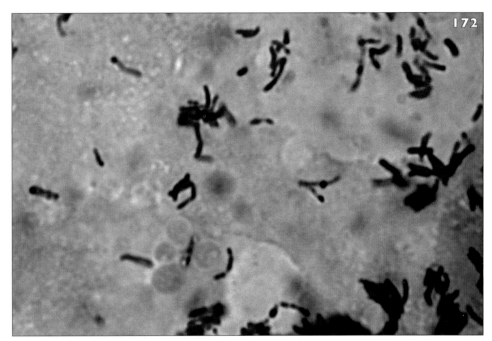

173 The structural components of the cell wall are important pathogenic properties of *Mycobacterium tuberculosis*.

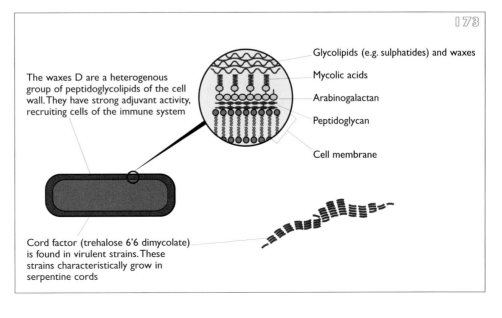

Pathogenesis

When a pathogen such as pneumococcus invades the lung, the infection is terminated when cells such as activated macrophages phagocytose the bacteria and destroy them. The ability of the macrophages to take up the bacteria is enhanced by certain acute phase proteins, complement, and antibodies, which neutralize the pathogenic potential of the encapsulated pneumococcus. In TB, a strong antibody response is mounted, but this plays no role in the disease process.

TB is a major problem for the immune system to deal with. This is due to the unusual components of the mycobacterial cell wall, which can interfere with cytokine activation of T cells and macrophages. Once inside the macrophage, mycobacteria inhibit the fusion of the phagosome and lysosome, and they can escape into the cytoplasm, thus evading the killing machinery of the macrophage.

It was stated in the introduction that nearly one-third of the world's population is infected with *Mycobacterium tuberculosis*, but clearly only a minority have active disease. An outline of the process that occurs in most individuals exposed to the mycobacterium is shown in **174a**. Droplet-borne organisms are inhaled and settle in the alveoli of the lung. The bacteria are phagocytosed by alveolar macrophages, which at this stage are unable to kill the bacteria. The mycobacteria thus reproduce both in and outside macrophages, and as their numbers increase, they

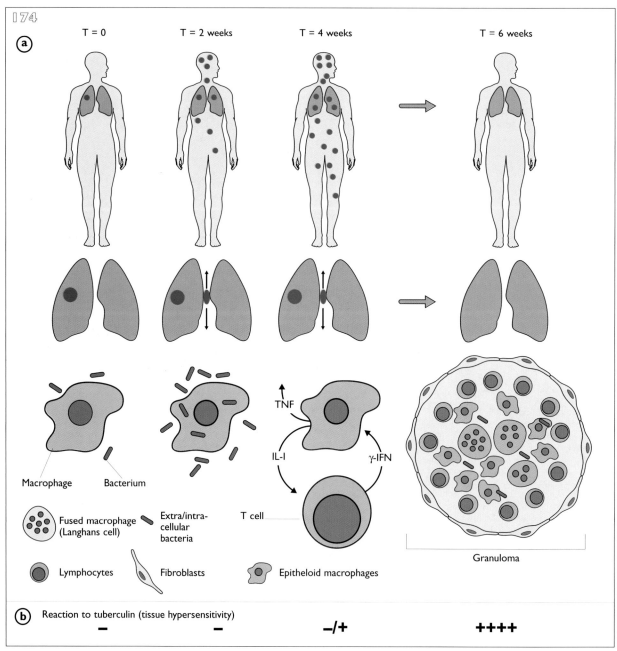

174 The first exposure to *Mycobacterium tuberculosis* usually results in a cell-mediated immunity response (delayed type hypersensitivity) which kills the bacteria.

spread, via infected macrophages, to the perihilar lymph nodes. Entering the blood the organisms are distributed throughout the body. This process takes several weeks and its length probably reflects the slow division rate of mycobacteria. After about 4 weeks, a cell-mediated immune response develops. Macrophages, activated by T cells, now contain high enough concentrations of enzymes and other metabolites that enable them to destroy the bacteria inside them. These activated macrophages are called epitheloid cells, which are organized in a structure called a granuloma. In the centre they fuse as multinucleate giant cells or Langhans cells. T cells and fibroblasts surround this effective killing machine. The whole process of cooperation between the T cells and macrophages and the degree of macrophage killing activity is tightly controlled by cell-to-cell contact and cytokines. The end result is the termination of the infection at all sites in the body that the organism has reached. This is a successful outcome. However, it is recognized that a few dormant bacteria may survive in macrophages for decades. These bacteria have the potential to cause reactivated disease many years later.

The development of the cell-mediated response in TB is also referred to as the delayed type hypersensitivity (DTH) response, which can be identified several weeks after infection by the Mantoux and Heaf tests (**174b**). Injection of purified protein derivative (PPD), an extract of boiled bacteria, into the dermis of the skin incites a local inflammatory response in those individuals who have a CMI response to the organism. The Heaf and Mantoux tests can be used to identify those individuals who have been infected.

A poor outcome of infection at primary exposure, in reactivated disease, or re-infection, depends on many factors but central to this is some compromise of the cell-mediated immune system. It is thus not surprising that immunosuppression, such as that arising from HIV infection and the use of steroids, pushes the infection towards the poorer outcome. Malnutrition and a very young age are other predisposing features. This emphasizes the fact that the ability to kill this difficult organism relies on a fully functioning and integrated cell-mediated immune system. There may also be genetic based differences in the ability of macrophages to kill the organism. There are some strains of mice whose macrophages are more effective killers of mycobacteria than those of other strains. It is possible that ethnic groups exposed to TB for thousands of years, such as the Caucasians, have macrophages that can deal with the organism more effectively than races from Africa and Asia who have only been exposed to the organism in recent times.

The 'good' outcome of infection, outlined above, is shown in comparison with a 'poor' outcome in **175a, b**. In the 'poor' situation, the degree of hypersensitivity is also high. As the

175 (a) The end result of a good outcome is effective organization in a granuloma. **(b)** A poor outcome arises as a result of some defect in the cell-mediated response.

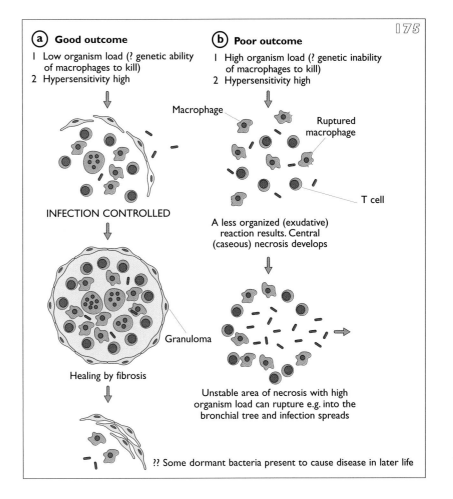

175

(a) Good outcome
1 Low organism load (? genetic ability of macrophages to kill)
2 Hypersensitivity high

(b) Poor outcome
1 High organism load (? genetic inability of macrophages to kill)
2 Hypersensitivity high

Macrophage

Ruptured macrophage

T cell

INFECTION CONTROLLED

A less organized (exudative) reaction results. Central (caseous) necrosis develops

Granuloma

Healing by fibrosis

Unstable area of necrosis with high organism load can rupture e.g. into the bronchial tree and infection spreads

?? Some dormant bacteria present to cause disease in later life

cell-mediated immune system is compromised for whatever reason, effective killing is not achieved and the organism numbers become high. The problem is exacerbated by the fact that cell wall components of mycobacteria act as adjuvants, directly attracting T cells and macrophages to the site of the infection. Uncontrolled lysis of macrophages releases large amounts of enzymes and metabolites that destroy the local tissue, leading to caseous necrosis. In the lung, areas of caseous necrosis are unstable and liquefy into adjacent areas. Cavities form, and when these fuse and break down, necrotic material laden with organisms spreads to other parts of the lung. The individual coughing up this material is the source of mycobacteria that others inhale.

Two broad types of clinical disease can be defined. Primary TB occurs following the initial exposure to the organism and secondary or reactivated disease occurs years later. An outline of infection and disease over time is shown in **176a, b**. If the outcome to the primary infection is favourable, the resulting cell-mediated response controls the infection wherever the organism is in the body. If the outcome is unfavourable, growth of the organism is not controlled and primary disease may manifest. In the hilar lymph nodes, inflammation can be significant, especially in young children, resulting in compression of the bronchi with symptoms of cough and stridor. Organisms seeding the meninges from the blood can give rise to meningitis. If a granuloma in the lung ruptures into the pleural space, the resulting hypersensitivity reaction results in a pleural effusion. Miliary TB is a manifestation of disseminated primary disease and derives its name from the numerous 'millet seed' sized lesions seen on chest X-ray. With one form of miliary disease, the patient can have meningitis and a septic or typhoidal clinical presentation.

When the primary infection is controlled, organisms can reside in tissue for many years where they have the potential to reactivate. Reactivation or secondary disease probably occurs as a consequence of an individual's CMI waning and dormant bacteria then reproduce to

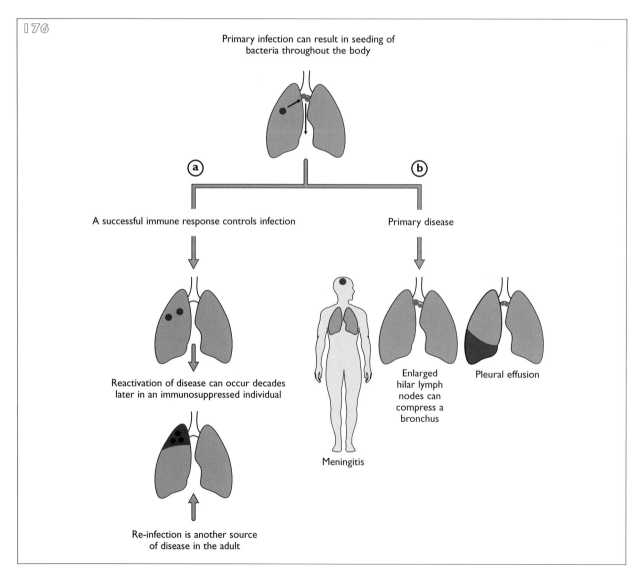

176 During primary infection the organism can spread to all organ systems. (**a**) The optimum outcome of the hypersensitivity response is control of the organism at all sites. (**b**) During primary infection stage, clinical disease such as meningitis and pleural effusion can occur.

overwhelm the now compromised defences. Reactivated disease often occurs in the upper, well-oxygenated lobes of the lung. Inability to control the infection leads to the breakdown of lesions, which fuse and develop into cavities of a size that can be seen on the chest X-ray. It is important to appreciate that reactivation is probably the likely mechanism of disease in older patients in areas where the incidence of TB is low. In areas where the incidence is high, re-infection is the more likely mechanism. Here again it will be the immuno-compromised patient who is likely to develop active disease following re-infection.

Active TB is a chronic infection centred on the cell-mediated immune response. Cytokines play an essential role in its pathogenesis, and systemic symptoms such as weight loss, fever, and night sweats, plus repair by fibrosis, are all features of the disease. The CRP and ESR are raised in these patients due to the chronic release of acute phase proteins by the liver.

Diagnosis

For any patient presenting with a history of fever, weight loss, night sweats, and cough, pulmonary TB must be considered. A characteristic chest X-ray and a positive ZN stain on expectorated sputum can confirm the diagnosis. It is important to remember that TB can arise in any organ. The frequency of involvement of various organs and sites and the specimens to collect are shown in **177**.

Infection control must be considered at this stage of diagnosis. It is essential that a confirmed or suspected case of 'open' pulmonary TB is nursed in a side room. These rooms should have a negative pressure ventilation system in order to reduce the organism load in the immediate environment of the patient, and minimize the chance of any spread to other patients and staff. This is of particular importance when considering the patient with MDR-TB.

In the microbiology laboratory both the ZN stain and the auramine stain are used. Auramine is a fluorescent dye that binds to cell wall components of mycobacteria and as

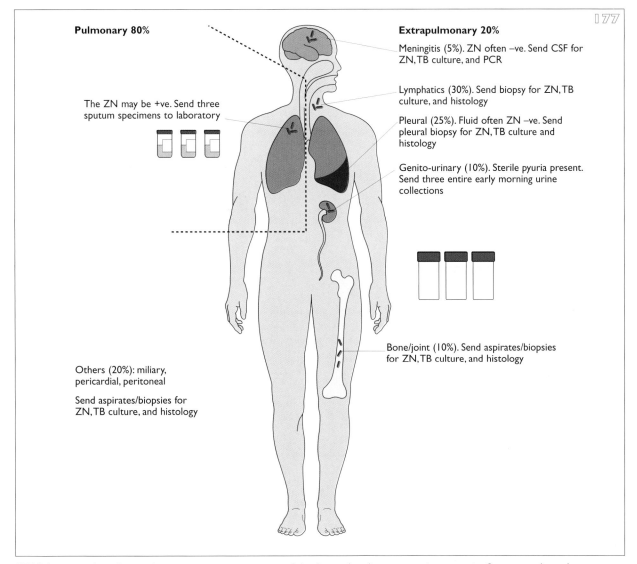

Pulmonary 80%

The ZN may be +ve. Send three sputum specimens to laboratory

Others (20%): miliary, pericardial, peritoneal

Send aspirates/biopsies for ZN, TB culture, and histology

Extrapulmonary 20%

Meningitis (5%). ZN often –ve. Send CSF for ZN, TB culture, and PCR

Lymphatics (30%). Send biopsy for ZN, TB culture, and histology

Pleural (25%). Fluid often ZN –ve. Send pleural biopsy for ZN, TB culture and histology

Genito-urinary (10%). Sterile pyuria present. Send three entire early morning urine collections

Bone/joint (10%). Send aspirates/biopsies for ZN, TB culture, and histology

177 Pulmonary tuberculosis is the most common presentation of the disease, but disease may arise at any site. Some examples and specimens to be collected are shown here.

it is more sensitive than the ZN stain, it is useful for screening large numbers of smears. Auramine-positive smears are then confirmed with the ZN stain.

An outline of the laboratory analysis of specimens is shown in **178**. Sputum specimens are decontaminated with sodium hydroxide to inactivate other bacterial contaminants. As mycobacteria are relatively hardy organisms, they resist this decontamination process. After neutralization of the alkaline step, sputum samples and all other specimens are centrifuged in order to concentrate any mycobacteria present. The centrifuged deposit is then used to inoculate media such as Lowenstein Jensen (LJ). Mycobacteria only divide every 15–20 hours or so, and thus the time taken to produce visible growth is slow in comparison to other bacteria. Inoculated agar 'slopes' are thus examined weekly for at least 6 weeks.

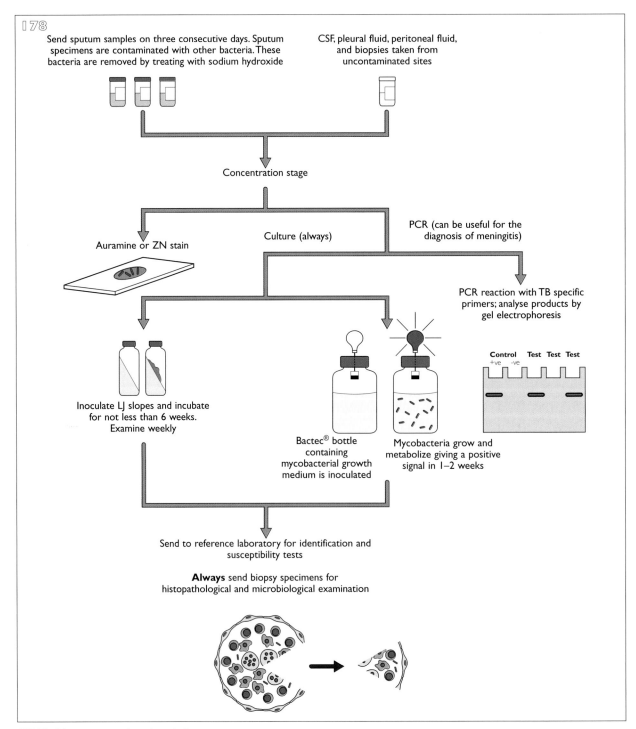

178 The laboratory tests for tuberculosis.

In order to circumvent this slow process, 'rapid' liquid culture systems are now available. In one such system, specimens are inoculated into media containing radioactive palmitate. Mycobacteria use this lipid as a substrate and the radioactive carbon dioxide appearing in the gas phase is detected. Other non-radioactive rapid systems are also available, where fluorescent sensors detect oxygen quenching in the liquid medium. On average it takes about 3–4 weeks before growth is seen on solid LJ medium, compared to 1–2 weeks in rapid liquid culture. Isolates of mycobacteria are usually sent to a reference laboratory where full identification and susceptibility tests are done. The antibiotics usually tested are INH, RIF, PZA, and ethambutol.

Rapid diagnosis by PCR can also be used, where specific sequences of the DNA, such as insertion sequence IS 1669, are amplified and separated by agar gel electrophoresis. The PCR is available in reference laboratories and its use may be restricted to situations where rapid diagnosis is important, for example in suspected TB meningitis. Histopathological examination of any tissue biopsy must always be considered. Organisms may not be seen when the tissue is prepared in the medical microbiology laboratory, but histology can identify the typical granuloma, and acid-fast organisms may be seen in stained sections.

If a biopsy is taken for histology and TB is a consideration, it is essential that some of the sample is also sent to the microbiology laboratory. If the entire specimen is fixed in formalin, the opportunity to grow, identify the organism, and determine its susceptibility profile will be lost.

Treatment

The usual treatment for pulmonary TB is the triple therapy regime consisting of INH, RIF, and PZA. The structure and known mode of action of these agents is shown in **179a**. These agents are taken once a day. After 2 months, INH and RIF are continued for a further 4 months. In the case of meningitis for example, INH and RIF are given for 9 months. The triple therapy regime is suitable for patients of Caucasian origin, especially where the incidence of drug resistance is low. The addition of ethambutol as a fourth agent is recommended when the patient comes from an area where the incidence of drug resistant organism is higher, e.g. patients from the ethnic minorities as well as recent immigrants and refugees.

It is essential that the patient on anti-TB treatment is closely monitored. Compliance over a long period is a problem, and in many places directly observed therapy (DOT) is practised. Here the patient reports daily to a clinic and is observed taking the tablets. Toxicity is another issue. INH, RIF, and PZA are all potentially hepatotoxic, and base line LFT should be performed before treatment is started. It is important to have an index of suspicion and the patient with nausea and right upper quadrant tenderness must have liver functions checked (**179b**). A bilirubin of >60 µmol/L and raised levels of aspartate transaminase (AST) and alanine transaminase (ALT) should prompt assessment of the patient and the discontinuation of the agents. An alternative combination in the setting of deranged LFT is ethambutol and

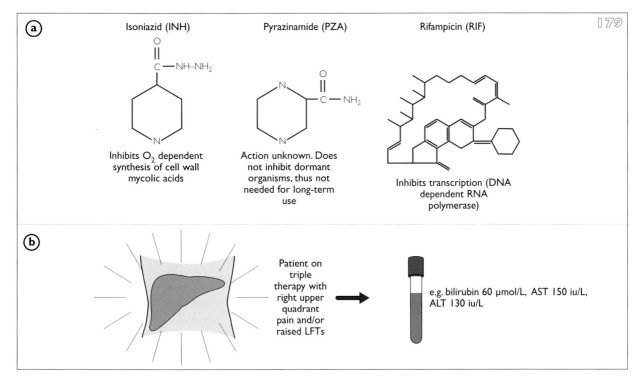

179 (a) The three front line agents commonly used to treat tuberculosis. **(b)** Drug-induced hepatitis needs to be checked for. (ALT: alanine transaminase; AST: aspartate transaminase.)

streptomycin, bearing in mind that both these agents can be nephrotoxic.

Isolates of *Mycobacterium tuberculosis* resistant to one or more agent are not uncommon. INH resistance is the most common and MDR-TB isolates resistant to INH and RIF have been found. Other agents used to treat these difficult cases include ciprofloxacin, clarithromycin, and the aminoglycoside amikacin.

It is essential that any patient treated for TB is referred to the chest physician, who has the experience and knowledge to determine the correct management. The chest physicians liase with public health departments to ensure that there is compliance of treatment, and that contacts are traced. If the treatment regime is correct the patient should be non-infectious within 2 weeks and may then be nursed on the open ward if they need to remain in hospital. Clearly resolution of symptoms over a number of days is reassuring. The patient who still remains unwell after this period with no sign of improvement must be reassessed. The possibility that the patient is not taking the drugs or that the organism is resistant must be considered. The reference laboratory performing the susceptibility tests should relay the results of any drug resistant isolate promptly.

Public health issues

The BCG (Bacillus Calmette–Guerin) vaccine and the tuberculin skin tests are also used in the management of TB. The Mantoux and Heaf skin tests are used to assess an individual's hypersensitivity to *Mycobaterium tuberculosis*.

Skin tests using PPD can be used for screening programs to determine the annual infection rate in a community. They can aid diagnosis or they can be used to identify the status of individuals who are contacts of a case. The different reactions to PPD are then used to decide whether a contact needs BCG vaccination, chemoprophylaxis or further clinical investigation.

The BCG vaccine is a live attenuated strain of *Mycobacterium bovis* and its use and efficacy throughout the world is variable. In the United Kingdom, recommendations for its use in individuals who do not have a positive tuberculin skin test, include health care workers who work in high risk clinical and laboratory settings, prison staff, contacts of an individual with active pulmonary disease and immigrants from areas of the world where the incidence of TB is high.

With the Mantoux test, PPD is injected into the dermis of the anterior forearm (**180a**). The degree of hypersensitivity is determined by examining the injection site 48–72 hours later (**180b**). While previous BCG vaccination can give a positive result, the response to PPD is most useful in patients who have not been vaccinated. A reaction of >15 mm identifies individuals who are certainly infected and who need further investigation, and this would at least include a CXR. Those individuals who have no reaction to PPD have not come into contact with the organism, or they could be in the early stages of primary exposure, before DTH develops. In the setting of exposure to a case of TB, it is these latter individuals who could be offered prophylaxis with INH for 6 months.

An outline of public health actions that should be taken when the index case is diagnosed as having active pulmonary TB is shown in **181**. For the purposes of this example, none of the five contacts of the case has had BCG

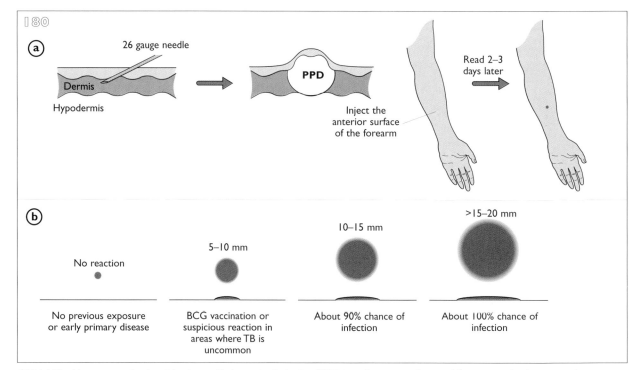

180 (a) The Mantoux test involves injecting purified protein derivative (PPD) into the anterior forearm. The extent of induration is then recorded. **(b)** The size of the reaction to PPD is used in management of contacts.

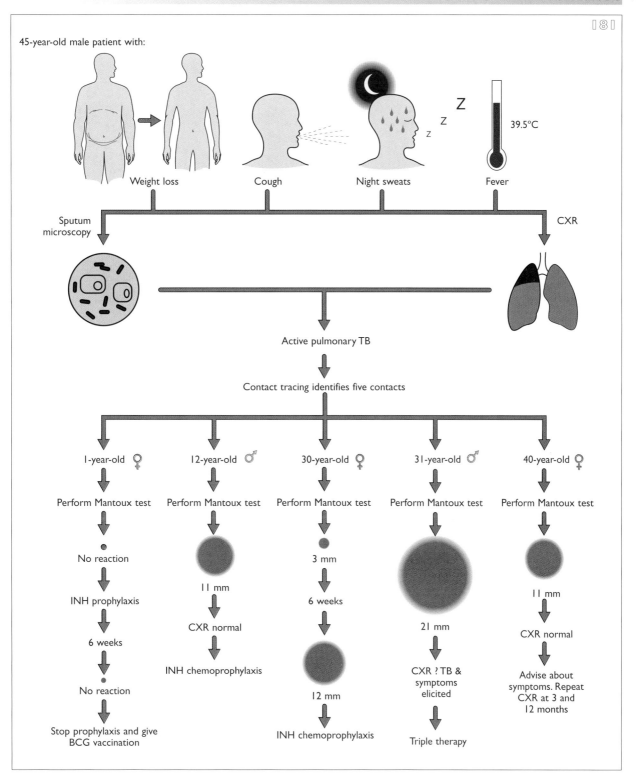

181 A 45-year-old patient is identified as having active pulmonary tuberculosis. None of the contacts have had the Bacillus Calmette-Guerin vaccine; examples of the management of such contacts are shown here.

vaccine. The results of the tuberculin test and further investigations such as chest X-ray determine the course of action for each contact. In the case shown in **181** there are two children under 16 years of age. The 1-year-old child had no response to tuberculin test, and in view of the possibility of serious primary disease at this age INH prophylaxis is given. Six weeks later the skin test is repeated and is still negative. It is reasonable to assume that this child has not been infected. The INH can stop and BCG vaccination is given. The 12-year-old child has a suspicious reaction. A normal chest X-ray rules out the likelihood of pulmonary disease and INH prophylaxis is given.

The logic here is that the single agent will help the CMI response to control infection at this stage. The 30-year-old adult's tuberculin test changes from 3 mm to 12 mm over the 6 week period, indicating recent infection and developing CMI. INH prophylaxis is appropriate here as well. The 31-year-old adult has a florid hypersensitivity reaction, and further questioning elicits the symptoms of TB, which is confirmed by chest X-ray and the examination of sputum. The 40-year-old adult has a positive Mantoux and normal chest X-ray. She has clearly been infected in the past and is given advice about symptoms and the need for a repeat chest X-ray 3 and 12 months later.

An essential aspect of the control of TB is the notification of any case to the public health authorities. A patient may be started empirically on TB treatment as a 'trial of treatment' when there are no positive results. These patients must also be notified to the public health authorities who will follow-up the family and other contacts that may identify cases of hitherto unknown active TB.

Comment

The BTS guidelines for the control and prevention of tuberculosis can be found in the following publication:

Joint Tuberculosis Committee (2000). Control and prevention of tuberculosis in the United Kingdom: code of practice 2000. *Thorax* **55**: 887–901.

Two articles that give a useful insight into the management of outbreaks of tuberculosis are listed below:

Kline SE (1995). Outbreak of tuberculosis among regular patrons of a neighbourhood bar. *New England Journal of Medicine* **333**: 222–7.

Small PM (1993). Exogenous reinfection with multidrug-resistant *Mycobacterium tuberculosis* in patients with advanced HIV infection. *New England Journal of Medicine* **328**: 1137–44.

9 Infections of the Central Nervous System

Introduction

The brain and spinal cord are protected by the skull and spinal column. Three connective tissue layers, the pia mater, arachnoid mater, and dura mater separate the nervous tissue from bone (**182**). Between the first two layers of connective tissue in the subarachnoid space is the cerebrospinal fluid (CSF), which acts as a shock absorber. It is produced by the choroid plexus of the ventricles, exiting by the foramina of Luschka and Magendie, and then circulates around the brain and spinal cord (**183**). CSF is reabsorbed by the arachnoid granulations, which extend into the superior sagittal sinus, one of the great vessels draining the brain. A blood–brain barrier is well recognized, and consists of capillary endothelial cells resting on a basement membrane. The tight junction between these cells is such that many constituents of the plasma are unable to cross into the CSF under normal circumstances.

182 The various connective tissue layers that surround the brain and spinal cord. The subarachnoid space contains the cerebrospinal fluid.

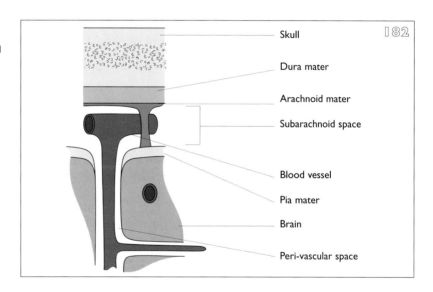

183 Cerebrospinal fluid is produced by the choroid plexus in the ventricles. It exits the ventricular system by the foraminae of Luschka and Magendie and circulates over the surface of the brain and spinal cord. (Modified, with permission from Lindsay KW *et al.* (1986) *Neurology and Neurosurgery Illustrated*. Churchill Livingstone, pp. 565.)

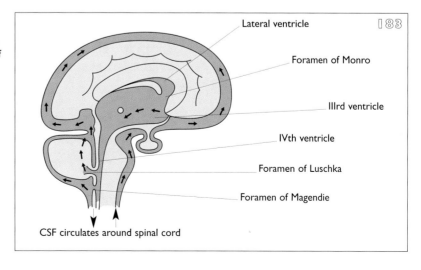

Any pathology in the brain which increases intracranial pressure can have disastrous consequences, as the bony skull and fibrous supports of the brain do not allow room for any significant expansion. Brain swelling thus leads to compression, herniation of the brain, and brain cell death. The pathological process that occurs, for example in meningitis, is outlined in **184a–c**. Here a simplified 'brain' is shown enclosed in the skull. The inflammatory response in the subarachnoid space and release of cytokines results in loosening of the tight junctions between vascular endothelial cells. This allows albumin into the CSF, producing vasogenic oedema. Toxic substances from bacteria and neutrophils, and a compromise in the supply of oxygen and nutrients to brain cells, results in cytotoxic oedema. Vasogenic and cytotoxic oedema both contribute to brain swelling which obstructs the outflow of CSF from the ventricles. The pressure behind this obstruction forces fluid from the CSF into the interstitial compartment, compounding the swelling. If medical intervention is not prompt, brain damage or brain death are likely outcomes.

Organisms can reach the brain and spinal cord by a number of routes. The brain has an extensive arterial and venous system (**185a, b**). The arterial system can transport organisms in septic emboli from distant sites of infection such as a lung abscess or an infected heart valve. Bacteria such as meningococcus enter the blood

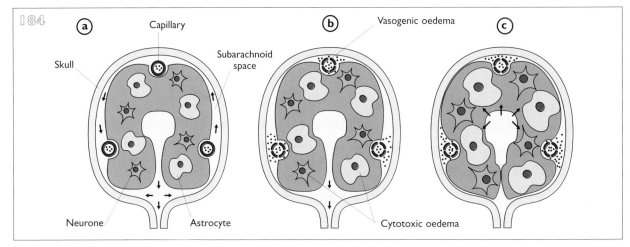

184 (**a**) The 'normal' brain. (**b**) Inflammatory conditions such as meningitis result in vasogenic and cytotoxic oedema. (**c**) Obstruction of cerebrospinal fluid outflow forces fluid into the interstitium, causing interstitial oedema.

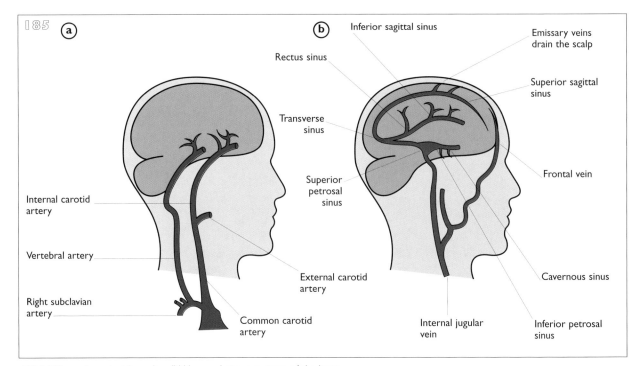

185 (**a**) The major arterial supplies. (**b**) Venous drainage systems of the brain.

from the nasopharynx and reach the brain via the arterial system; if they manage to enter the CSF, meningitis is the likely result. Septic thrombophlebitis can occur in the main venous structures associated with the brain, such as the cavernous sinus, venous sinuses, and the tributaries of the jugular veins. Within the skull lie the nasal sinuses and mastoid air spaces, separated in places from the brain by thin bone. Infection here may erode through the bone into the brain. Some sources of bacteria that cause meningitis or a brain abscess are shown in **186a, b**.

The array of infective conditions of the central nervous system is impressive, as is their clinical presentation. Meningitis, encephalitis, brain abscess, subdural and epidural abscesses, and cavernous sinus thrombosis are examples. Clinical symptoms may be non-specific, such as fever, headache, and vomiting, or there may be a specific neurological deficit caused by a lesion at a particular site in the brain. Encephalitis due to herpes simplex virus (HSV) may manifest as unusual behaviour, characteristic of the replication of the virus within cells of the temporal lobe. Toxins are responsible for botulism and tetanus. Guillain-Barré syndrome is a polyneuropathy, the commonest infectious cause being campylobacter gastroenteritis.

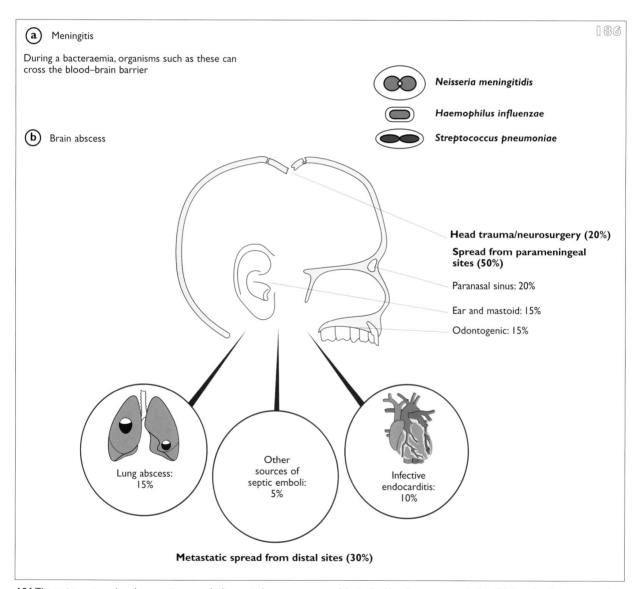

186 The main routes whereby organisms reach the central nervous system: (**a**) via the blood to cause meningitis; (**b**) from local sites or septic emboli to initiate a brain abscess.

The range of organisms that can cause disease in the central nervous system is vast. In addition to the bacteria detailed in this chapter, fungi, viruses, protozoa, and eucaryotic parasites are all able to cause infection. Examples include the yeast *Cryptococcus neoformans*, an important cause of meningitis in AIDS patients, and viruses such as HSV, varicella zoster virus (VZV), and the enteroviruses. When cysts of the pork tapeworm *Taenia solium* settle in the brain, neurocysticercosis arises; the resulting inflammation can cause epilepsy which may be the first manifestation of this infection.

Organisms

A list of bacteria to consider in various clinical settings is shown in **187a–d**. Disease can be caused by true exogenous pathogens such as *Mycobacterium tuberculosis* or *Listeria monocytogenes*. Listeria can be acquired from eating food contaminated with the organism. Preterm neonates or those subjected to prolonged labour are at risk of invasive disease, including meningitis, by group B streptococcus, acquired from the maternal vaginal flora during delivery. Pathogens such as *Neisseria meningitidis*, *Haemophilus influenzae* b, and pneumococcus can be members of the 'normal' flora of the nasopharynx.

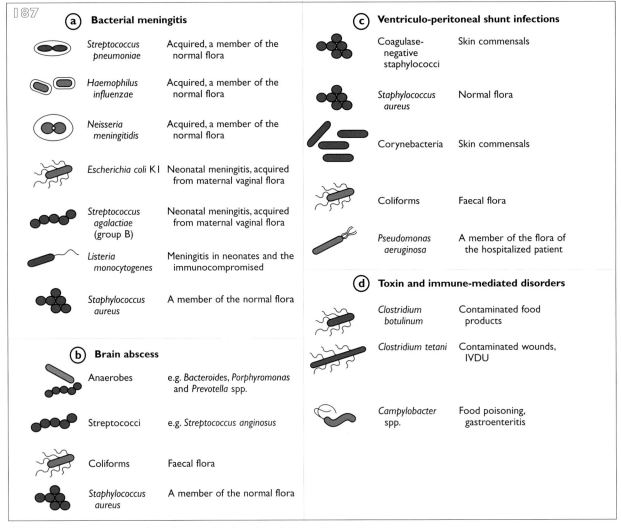

187

(a) Bacterial meningitis

	Streptococcus pneumoniae	Acquired, a member of the normal flora
	Haemophilus influenzae	Acquired, a member of the normal flora
	Neisseria meningitidis	Acquired, a member of the normal flora
	Escherichia coli K1	Neonatal meningitis, acquired from maternal vaginal flora
	Streptococcus agalactiae (group B)	Neonatal meningitis, acquired from maternal vaginal flora
	Listeria monocytogenes	Meningitis in neonates and the immunocompromised
	Staphylococcus aureus	A member of the normal flora

(b) Brain abscess

	Anaerobes	e.g. *Bacteroides*, *Porphyromonas* and *Prevotella* spp.
	Streptococci	e.g. *Streptococcus anginosus*
	Coliforms	Faecal flora
	Staphylococcus aureus	A member of the normal flora

(c) Ventriculo-peritoneal shunt infections

	Coagulase-negative staphylococci	Skin commensals
	Staphylococcus aureus	Normal flora
	Corynebacteria	Skin commensals
	Coliforms	Faecal flora
	Pseudomonas aeruginosa	A member of the flora of the hospitalized patient

(d) Toxin and immune-mediated disorders

	Clostridium botulinum	Contaminated food products
	Clostridium tetani	Contaminated wounds, IVDU
	Campylobacter spp.	Food poisoning, gastroenteritis

187a–d A list of more common bacteria to consider in various clinical settings.

The normal flora itself is also important. The patient with chronic suppurative lung disease arising from aspiration of oral bacteria may develop a brain abscess following an embolic episode from the lung. Ventriculo-peritoneal shunt infections are usually caused by skin organisms such as the coagulase-negative staphylococci, which can contaminate the shunt at the time of insertion.

Pathogenesis
Meningitis

Meningococcus and *Haemophilus influenzae* b are members of the normal flora and, under certain conditions, enter the blood. This ability to enter the blood depends on various host and organism factors, as shown in **188a, b**. It is probable that meningococcus loses

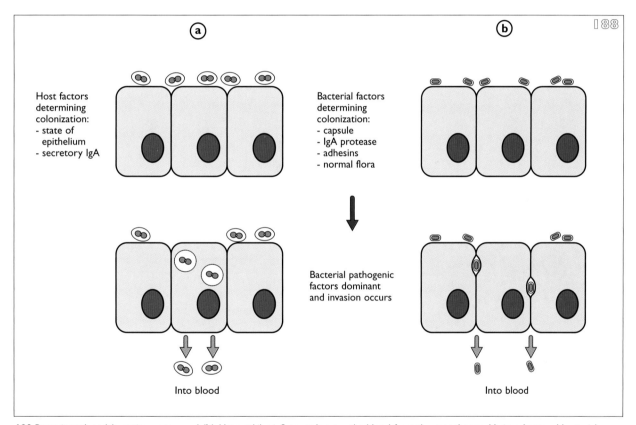

188 Bacteria such as (**a**) meningococcus and (**b**) *Haemophilus influenzae* b enter the blood from the nasopharynx. Various host and bacterial factors influence the process.

its capsule in order to be effectively transported across the epithelium. Haemophilus appears to cross the epithelium by traversing the junction between cells. Once in the blood these bacteria must be encapsulated in order to reduce any chance of being phagocytosed. In the capillary system of the brain, bacteria can attach to the endothelium by adhesins. A few organisms enter the subarachnoid space and the process of meningitis is initiated (**189–193**). These few bacteria initially have an advantage as CSF has low levels of complement and IgG.

An immune response is mounted and, via cytokines, expression of selectin and integrin proteins on the surface of endothelial cells and neutrophils occurs. Interaction between these proteins results in the margination of the neutrophils onto the endothelium. Loosening of the inter-cellular junction allows the neutrophils, albumin, and other plasma proteins to enter the CSF. The end result is the classic picture of bacterial meningitis, with large numbers of bacteria, neutrophils, and a raised protein. Metabolism of glucose by the white blood cells (WBCs) and bacteria results in a significant lowering of CSF glucose.

Brain abscess

Once bacteria enter the brain tissue, for example from an infected embolus lodged in a small vessel, a cerebritis will develop over a number of days as the inflammatory response attempts to control bacterial growth. Progression to a central area of necrosis results in an abscess, which becomes covered in a collagen capsule laid down by fibroblasts. Around this expanding abscess is a zone of tissue oedema and the whole structure exerts a mass effect, compressing the brain against its fibrous supports and the skull (**194a–c**). A lumbar puncture (LP) should not be done in these circumstances. Removing fluid from the subarachnoid space in the spine will increase the pressure difference between the brain and the cord, exacerbating any pressure effect. The resulting herniation of the brain can have disastrous consequences.

More centrally situated abscesses can rupture into the ventricles. The blood supply to the central white matter is less than elsewhere in the brain and the action of the fibroblasts in laying down the collagen capsule is compromised. The weaker medial side of the capsule can then rupture, releasing pus into the ventricles.

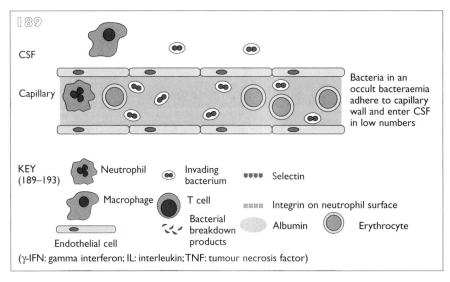

CSF

Capillary

Bacteria in an occult bacteraemia adhere to capillary wall and enter CSF in low numbers

KEY (189–193)

Neutrophil — Invading bacterium — Selectin

Macrophage — T cell — Integrin on neutrophil surface

Endothelial cell — Bacterial breakdown products — Albumin — Erythrocyte

(γ-IFN: gamma interferon; IL: interleukin; TNF: tumour necrosis factor)

189–193 A simplified outline of the stages that occur in meningococcal meningitis, which take place over a period of 12–24 hours: **189** Entry into the cerebrospinal fluid.

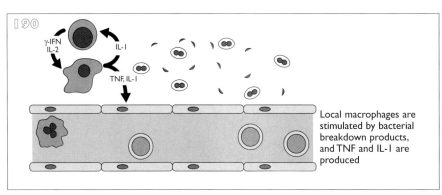

γ-IFN
IL-2

IL-1

TNF, IL-1

Local macrophages are stimulated by bacterial breakdown products, and TNF and IL-1 are produced

190 Stimulation of the immune response.

191 Margination of neutrophils.

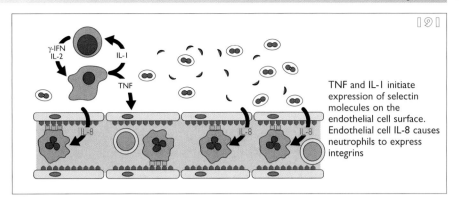

TNF and IL-1 initiate expression of selectin molecules on the endothelial cell surface. Endothelial cell IL-8 causes neutrophils to express integrins

192 Entry of neutrophils and albumin into the CSF.

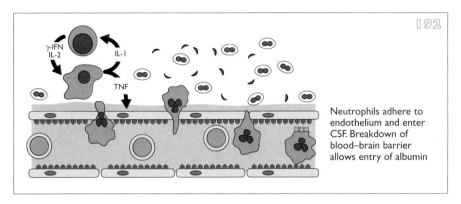

Neutrophils adhere to endothelium and enter CSF. Breakdown of blood–brain barrier allows entry of albumin

193 The last stage: entry of neutrophils and albumin into the CSF.

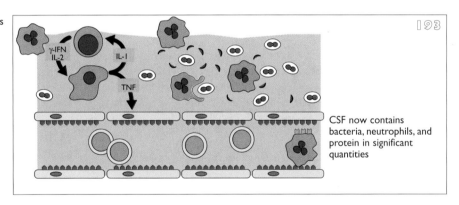

CSF now contains bacteria, neutrophils, and protein in significant quantities

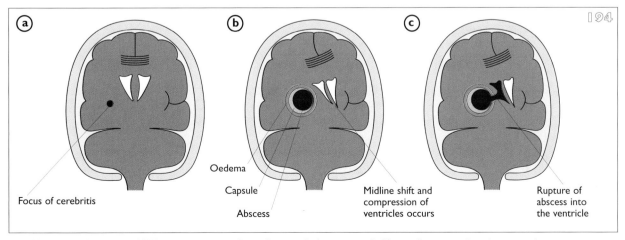

Focus of cerebritis

Oedema

Capsule

Abscess

Midline shift and compression of ventricles occurs

Rupture of abscess into the ventricle

194 (a) A focus of cerebritis. (b) This progresses to a brain abscess, which is surrounded by a collagen capsule and tissue oedema. (c) An abscess can rupture into the ventricle.

Subdural and extradural infections

Bacteria can enter both the subdural and extradural spaces (**195a–c**). In the subdural space, organisms can spread easily in the potential space between the arachnoid and dura mater. Extradural infections tend to be more localized because of fibrous attachments of the dura to the skull. Infections can also occur in relation to the spinal cord (**196a–d**). In both extradural and subdural infections, the mass effect at the site of the infection can give rise to compression of the spinal cord, which is a neurosurgical emergency.

Ventriculo-peritoneal shunt infections

Ventriculo-peritoneal shunts are inserted to relieve hydrocephalus. Non-communicating hydrocephalus may result from a congenital abnormality or it can be acquired. Fibrosis and subsequent blockage of the CSF outflow channels can develop as a result of an intraventricular haemorrhage in a premature neonate, or following bacterial ventriculitis. In order to relieve the hydrocephalus, a shunt is inserted into a ventricle, exits the skull, and via a subcutaneous route, drains CSF into the peritoneum. Organisms may be introduced at the time of operation and initiate shunt infection some time later. Usually skin bacteria such as coagulase-negative staphylococci are involved. Patients may present with a headache and low-grade fever, and may have symptoms and signs of peritonitis, indicating colonization of the shunt throughout its course (**197a–c**).

Tetanus

Clostridium tetani is a spore forming, motile gram-positive obligate anaerobe. The spore is very stable and can survive in soil and animal manure for years. Disease may arise in the elderly individual whose immunity has waned or in those who have never been vaccinated. When anaerobic conditions exist in a soft tissue injury, the spores germinate and the vegetative cells produce the toxin. An outline of the action of the toxin is shown in **198a, b**. The active component enters the terminals of lower motor neurons, where it inhibits neurotransmitter release. It then travels in a retrograde direction to reach the cell bodies and terminals of inhibitory cells in the CNS. By irreversibly inhibiting the action of glycine and GABA-mediated inhibitory neurons, the motor neurons are left relatively unaffected and spastic paralysis occurs.

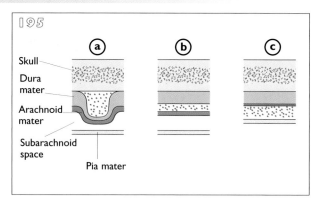

195 Infection in the connective tissue layers surrounding the brain and spinal cord can give rise to: (**a**) extradural; (**b**) subdural; and (**c**) subarachnoid (meningeal) infections.

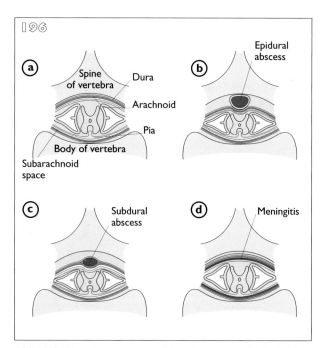

196 (**a**) Outline of the structure of the spinal column. (**b**) Epidural, (**c**) subdural, and (**d**) subarachnoid (meningeal) infections.

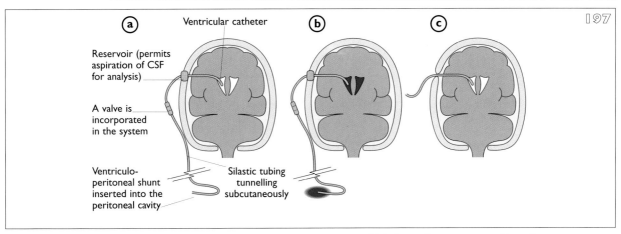

197 (**a**) A ventriculo-peritoneal shunt drains cerebrospinal fluid into the peritoneum. (**b**) A shunt infection can extend from the ventricles to the peritoneum. (**c**) Usually the ventricular portion is externalized.

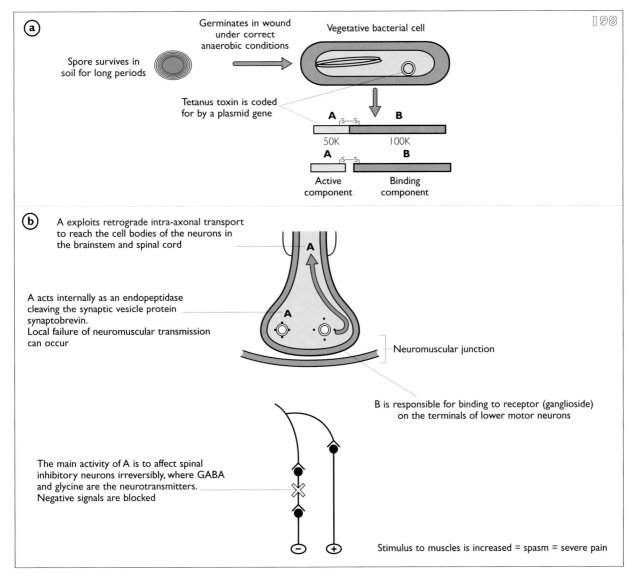

198 Some features of (**a**) the tetanus toxin and (**b**) its mode of action. (GABA: gamma amino-n-butyric acid.)

Botulism

Botulism is caused by *Clostridium botulinum*. This disease is a true intoxication. The bacterial spores survive cooking and germinate in food that is stored incorrectly; the vegetative cells produce toxin. When the food is consumed the toxin is absorbed into the blood. The active component of the toxin inhibits the release of acetylcholine at the neuromuscular junction and flaccid paralysis arises (**199a, b**).

Guillain-Barré syndrome

This condition is also termed acute post-infectious polyneuropathy and is precipitated by a number of infectious agents including mycoplasma and EBV. The most common infective cause is considered to be due to certain strains of campylobacter that have the surface O lipopolysaccharide 19. Following gastroenteritis, an immune-mediated process acts on the axons and myelin sheath leading to sensory, motor, and autonomic defects. Progressive motor dysfunction can lead to respiratory compromise and the patient may need to be ventilated. Mild disease has a good prognosis, while patients who need ventilation may have life-long disability.

Diagnosis

The diagnosis of infection in the central nervous system may be obvious. The patient with fever, headache, vomiting, photophobia, and the typical rash of meningococcal infection has meningococcal sepsis and meningitis. On other occasions, patients may present with abnormal behaviour which may be the first indication of a brain abscess.

Radiological investigations such as computed tomography (CT) and magnetic resonance imaging (MRI) scans are an essential part of diagnosis and they can determine the degree of brain swelling in meningitis, as well as the size and site of a brain abscess. These procedures are also used to rule out mass lesions before a LP is conducted.

Laboratory diagnosis

The need to perform a LP may be different for various age groups. When meningitis is considered in young children, a LP may not be done and an antibiotic active against meningococcus, pneumococcus, and haemophilus would be prescribed. However, blood cultures should always be taken, and in the case of suspected meningococcal disease an EDTA blood sample should be collected for meningococcal PCR. In adults the need for LP to confirm the diagnosis may be more pressing. In addition to meningococcus and pneumococcus, other organisms such as listeria may be considered, and CSF for culture is important.

It is essential once CSF or pus from an abscess has been collected that it is sent to the laboratory promptly for microscopy and culture. In the case of the HIV patient with AIDS, an India ink stain of the CSF should be done for cryptococcus. The large capsule of these yeasts shows up clearly against the black background of the ink (**200**).

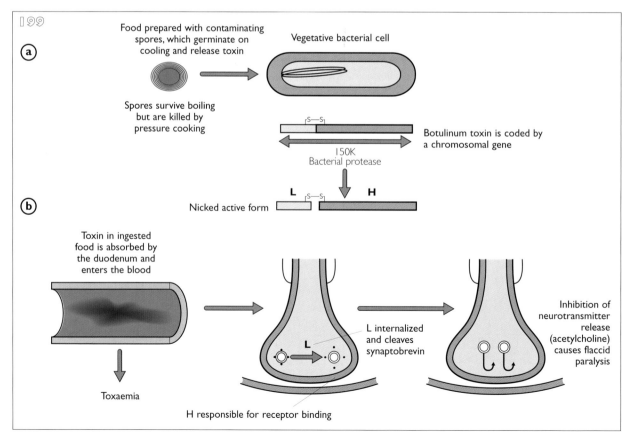

199 Some features of (**a**) the botulism toxin and (**b**) its mode of action.

It is usual to collect three samples of CSF; the first two are sent for protein and glucose determination and the third to the medical microbiology department. Microscopical and biochemical parameters used in the interpretation of CSF specimens are shown in **201**. The differentiation between normal CSF values and those representative of bacterial, viral, and tuberculous meningitis is often useful. In bacterial and tuberculous meningitis the protein is raised and the glucose low. Neutrophils are the predominant cell type in bacterial meningitis and monocytes in tuberculous meningitis. In viral meningitis a normal glucose and moderately raised protein in the setting of a lymphocytosis is the usual finding. Where relevant, CSF should be processed for viral culture and HSV and VZV PCR. It is always essential to consider TB, and rapid culture and PCR should be used in the appropriate clinical setting. Stains for mycobacteria are seldom positive in the setting of tuberculous meningitis.

CT scans are essential in the diagnosis of brain and other central nervous system abscesses. Scanning enables the neurosurgeon to visualize and enter the abscess to drain fluid, relieving intracranial pressure. The specimen obtained is vital for microbiological and histopathological examination. CT scans are also used to determine if an abscess is responding to treatment (**202a–c**).

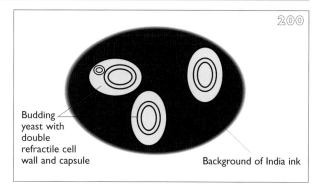

200

Budding yeast with double refractile cell wall and capsule

Background of India ink

200 The capsule of *Cryptococcus neoformans* shows up clearly when cerebrospinal fluid is stained with India ink.

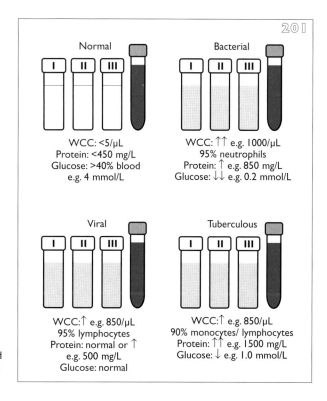

201

Normal

WCC: <5/μL
Protein: <450 mg/L
Glucose: >40% blood
e.g. 4 mmol/L

Bacterial

WCC: ↑↑ e.g. 1000/μL
95% neutrophils
Protein: ↑ e.g. 850 mg/L
Glucose: ↓↓ e.g. 0.2 mmol/L

Viral

WCC: ↑ e.g. 850/μL
95% lymphocytes
Protein: normal or ↑
e.g. 500 mg/L
Glucose: normal

Tuberculous

WCC: ↑ e.g. 850/μL
90% monocytes/ lymphocytes
Protein: ↑↑ e.g. 1500 mg/L
Glucose: ↓ e.g. 1.0 mmol/L

201 When collecting cerebrospinal fluid (CSF), three specimens should be taken, as well as serum for glucose determination. The features of a normal, bacterial, tuberculous and viral CSF are shown.

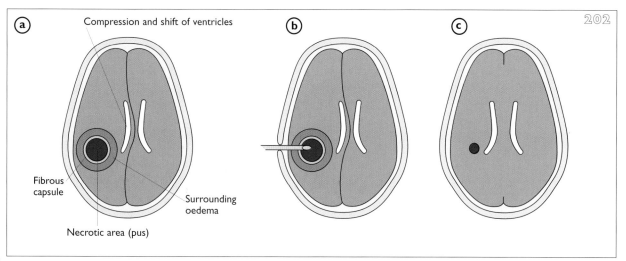

202

(a) Compression and shift of ventricles

Fibrous capsule

Necrotic area (pus)

Surrounding oedema

(b)

(c)

202 Computerized tomography scans are important in: (**a**) the diagnosis; (**b**) surgical intervention; (**c**) follow-up management of a brain abscess.

The diagnosis of tetanus and botulism is outlined in **203** and **204** respectively. Both are essentially clinical diagnoses, but in the case of botulism the toxin may be identified in blood and in suspected food. Guillain-Barré is also a clinical diagnosis. A recent history of campylobacter diarrhoea may be relevant and the presence of raised IgM and IgA antibodies to the organism is also of clinical use.

Treatment

Appropriate antibiotics to use are shown in **205a–d**. For 'community acquired' meningitis, pneumococcus, meningococcus and, in the unvaccinated child less than 5 years of age, *Haemophilus influenzae* b would be considered. The third generation cephalosporins cefotaxime or ceftriaxone are a good choice, as reliable levels are achieved in the CSF. Ceftriaxone is appealing as the regime for the adult patient is 2 g once a day. Depending on local susceptibility patterns, benzylpenicillin is also useful for meningococcus and pneumococcus; however, the regime of 1.2 g 3 hourly requires reliable venous access.

Benzylpenicillin or amoxycillin should always be included where *Listeria monocytogenes* is a consideration, for example in the neonate or immunocompromised patient. It should be noted with listeria and group B streptococcus that gentamicin is given with the β-lactam. Aminoglycosides are often included as a second agent in the setting of meningitis being caused by a gram-negative organism, even though the penetration of these agents into the CSF is not good. In certain circumstances the possible causative agent may include viruses such as HSV and VZV,

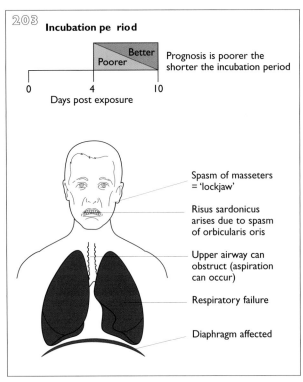

203 The diagnosis of tetanus is largely based on clinical evidence.

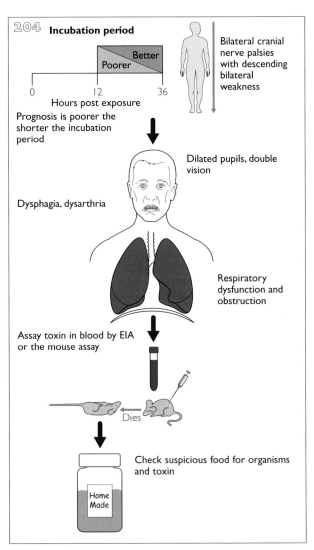

204 In addition to clinical evidence, the presence of botulism toxin can be confirmed in the blood of patients and in the likely food source, from where the organism can be isolated.

and an antiviral agent effective against herpes viruses, for example aciclovir, should be given at least until laboratory results are available. The length of therapy used in the treatment of bacterial meningitis ranges from 5–7 days for meningococcus to 2–3 weeks for listeria meningitis.

For a brain abscess a combination of penicillin, chloramphenicol or cefotaxime, and metronidazole is often used. Clindamycin and RIF together are useful substitutes for penicillin and metronidazole. These regimes can be modified once the results of bacteriological investigations are available, and specific bacteria can be targeted. Treatment is given for 4–6 weeks.

In ventriculo-peritoneal shunt infections, vancomycin, ceftazidime, and RIF can be used initially. Vancomycin and RIF give cover for gram-positive organisms, of which coagulase-negative staphylococci are the most important. It should be noted that RIF should not be given alone for gram-positive organisms as resistance can develop rapidly. Ceftazidime provides suitable gram-negative cover including that for pseudomonas. The regime can be tailored depending on the isolates obtained. Often most of the shunt has to be removed, with the part draining the ventricles being externalized (**197c**). This route can be used to give intraventricular vancomycin; the dose is usually 10 mg once a day.

For toxin-mediated disease, ventilatory support is the mainstay. With tetanus metronidazole or benzylpenicillin are given, and surgical debridement is essential. With Guillain-Barré, ventilatory support is needed when the respiratory muscles are affected.

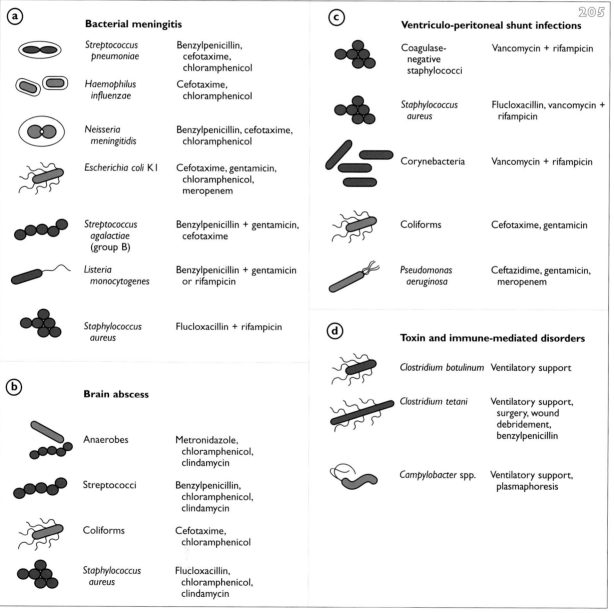

205a–d The bacteria associated with infections of the central nervous system, and examples of some antibiotics that can be used.

Public health issues

Invasive disease due to *Haemophilus influenzae* b was a significant cause of meningitis in children less than 5 years of age. With the advent of the Hib vaccine in the 1990s, this problem has largely been eliminated in countries where vaccination is practised; the introduction of the vaccine in the United Kingdom led to a dramatic drop in the number of cases (**206**). Vaccines for meningococcal types A and C have been available for years and a conjugated meningococcal C vaccine has now been introduced. There is no vaccine for serotype B, as the capsular material is not immunogenic. Research is being conducted to produce a vaccine using cell membrane proteins.

It is essential that any case of meningitis is notified to the public health authority or the CCDC. Any clinical or laboratory information that supports the identification of a particular organism must be relayed to these health care workers, in particular when meningococcus and haemophilus are involved, as tracing of family, school, university, and work contacts needs to be done. A useful 'rule' is the 4, 5, 7 rule where a contact who has had 4 hours of contact with the index case in any 5 days of the last week, needs to be considered for prophylaxis. Prophylaxis is given to reduce the overall carriage rate of the organisms in a defined population. Two antibiotics, RIF or ciprofloxacin are used in this situation. RIF induces liver enzymes, and this can affect the metabolism of agents such as the oral contraceptive. Relevant female individuals given RIF need to use an alternative form of contraception. For this reason ciprofloxacin as a single dose is appealing. Ceftriaxone as a single dose can be used in contacts that are pregnant. Where a vaccine is available for the organism isolated, for example the meningococcal C vaccine, it is recommended that the index case and contacts receive this.

Comment

Perhaps the most 'sensitive' specimen taken from a patient is CSF, for if procedures go wrong after collection there can be serious consequences. Three specimens should be collected with the first two being sent to the biochemistry department for protein and glucose determination, and the third to medical microbiology. It is important that the laboratories are contacted and informed about the specimens, in order that their arrival can be anticipated and to ensure that the correct tests are done. In addition to standard microbiological investigation, the specimen may also need investigation for TB, including PCR, and virological investigation. If there is limited material for the range of tests being considered, it is important to prioritize them with the medical microbiologist. If a subarachnoid haemorrhage is being investigated, it is essential that the three consecutive specimens be clearly labelled.

Although it is an article from 1992, the following reference provides useful background into the pathogenesis of bacterial meningitis:

Quagliarello V, Scheld MD (1992). Bacterial meningitis pathogenesis, pathology, and progress. *New England Journal of Medicine* **327**: 864–71.

The following article gives up-to-date information in the treatment of certain neurosurgical infections:

Brown EM (2000). The management of neurosurgical patients with postoperative bacterial or aseptic meningitis or external ventricular drain-associated ventriculitis. *British Journal of Neurology* **14**: 7–12.

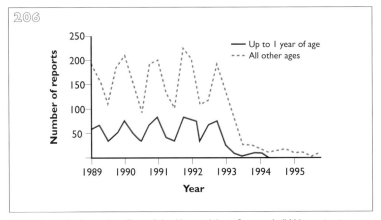

206 This graph shows the effect of the *Haemophilus influenzae* b (Hib) vaccine in reducing invasive haemophilus disease in England and Wales. (Modified, with permission from the Communicable Diseases Surveillance Centre, Colindale, London.)

10 Infections of the Eye

Introduction

Red eye is the most common disorder of the eye for which medical advice is sought. Conjunctivitis is the main entity encountered, and can be caused by infection, allergy, or chemical irritation. Infectious conjunctivitis can affect all age groups and resolution occurs in most cases following the application of topical antibiotics. Infection can occur in other parts of the eye, including the cornea, and the anterior and posterior chambers. Structures such as the orbit and cavernous sinuses can also be involved, and because of the proximity of these structures to the brain, life-threatening illness can occur. Any infection of the eye or its associated structures in the setting of pain and vision loss must be considered an emergency and the ophthalmologist needs to be consulted promptly. Infections of the eyelids, lacrymal glands, and nasolacrymal duct are also considered here. The gross anatomy of the eye and its adjacent structures are shown in **207**.

The main clinical entities considered here are conjunctivitis, keratitis (infection of the cornea) and endophthalmitis. While well known bacteria and viruses are involved in most infections, recent medical interventions have brought new agents onto the scene. The increased use of contact lenses and their cleaning in contaminated water has made the aquatic amoeba acanthamoeba a recognized cause of contact lens keratitis.

This contrasts with old diseases of the underdeveloped parts of the world. Trachoma is one example and is caused by the A, B, C serovars of *Chlamydia trachomatis*. It is estimated that 500 million people are affected, of whom 10 million are blinded. The organism is spread to the eye by hand and flies, and the chronic conjunctivitis that arises leads to scarring, corneal ulceration, and subsequent vision loss. In West, Central, and East Africa and parts of Central America, a scourge of the centuries has been river blindness, a disease that is estimated to occur in at least 20 million individuals. It is caused by the microfilaria of the parasite *Onchocerca volvulus*. This parasite is spread by the blood sucking simulid blackfly. The microfilarial stage of the parasite invades the anterior chamber of the eye, with corneal ulceration and fibrosis leading to blindness. The antiparasite drug ivermectin has had a significant effect in treating the condition in recent years.

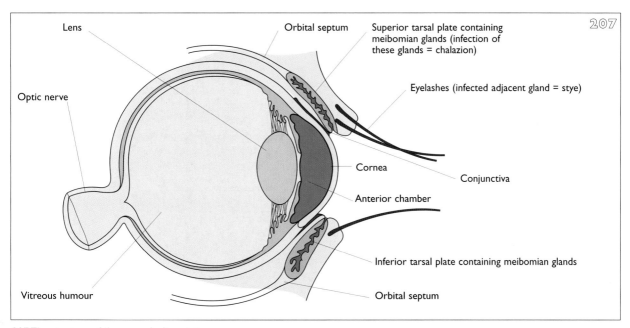

207 The structure of the eye and adjacent tissues.

Organisms

The organisms to consider in eye infections are shown in **208**. Certain viruses that cause conjunctivitis and keratitis are shown here as well.

Pathogenesis

Bacterial conjunctivitis is characterized by an inflamed red eye and associated discharge. Severe infection with significant eyelid oedema, extreme hyperaemia, and a profuse purulent discharge needs special mention. In this setting, bacteria such as *Neisseria gonorrhoea* and *Neisseria meningitidis* may be involved, and the massive release of lytic enzymes from dead and dying neutrophils

damage the cornea. Ulceration and perforation of the cornea here or following trauma, allows organisms to reach the anterior chamber and from there the vitreous humour, producing endophthalmitis (**209**). In the hospital setting, *Pseudomonas aeruginosa* can also initiate an aggressive keratitis, and can be of particular importance in the ICU patient who has had some superficial trauma to the cornea during their management. With keratitis there is usually some degree of pain and vision loss.

Endophthalmitis is infection of the vitreous humour (**210**). Organisms can enter the posterior eye following penetrating trauma, and soil-derived organisms such as *Bacillus cereus* need to be considered in these circum-

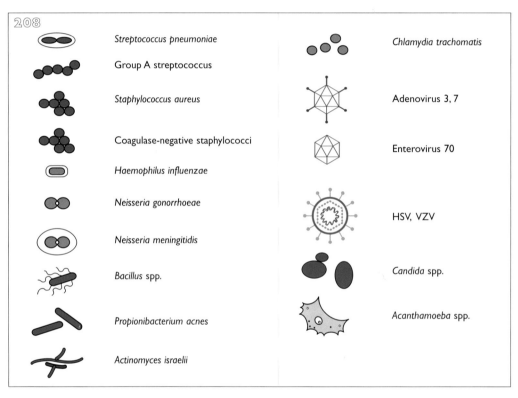

208 A list of some of the organisms to consider in infections of the eye.

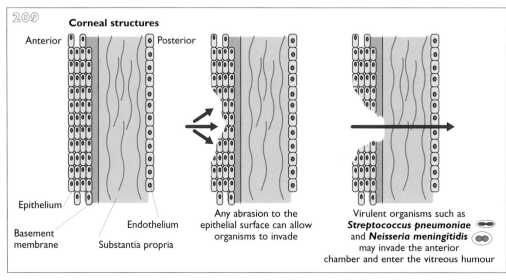

209 Abrasion of the epithelium allows organisms to invade the cornea and beyond.

stances. When penetrating injury is caused by plant material, some unusual bacteria may be isolated. In post-surgical endophthalmitis, bacteria such as coagulase-negative staphylococci are relevant. Organisms can also reach the vitreous humour via the blood and here an intra-vascular source such as endocarditis should be looked for.

Orbital cellulitis and cavernous sinus thrombosis may be difficult to distinguish from each other. Cellulitis usually arises as an extension of infection in a nasal sinus into the orbit. The tissue separating the orbit from the ethmoid air cells is thin, and can be easily damaged by trauma. Orbital cellulitis is associated with dark red skin over the eye,

headache, and fever. Pain associated with movement of the eye is also present, reflecting the inflammation in soft tissue that surrounds the eye within the orbital cavity. Because of the space restrictions within the cavity, forward displacement or proptosis of the eye occurs. Cavernous sinus thrombosis arises as a result of extension of thrombophlebitis of the facial veins. The patient is severely ill with headache, fevers, and chills. While the condition may be difficult to distinguish from orbital cellulitis, palsies of the IIIrd, IVth, and VIth cranial nerves, and bilateral signs may be helpful in the diagnosis. The main structures of the cavernous sinus are shown in **211**.

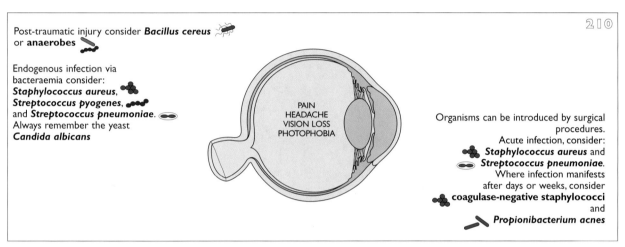

210 Organisms can reach the posterior chamber of the eye by three main routes, to cause endophthalmitis.

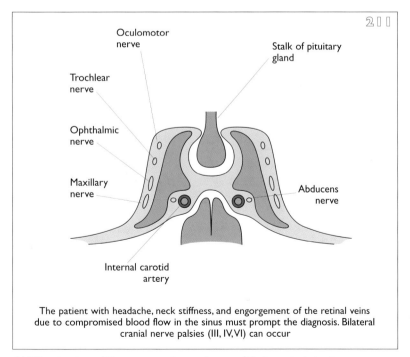

211 The structure of the cavernous sinus and some of the important structures that lie in it.

Eyelid abscesses such as a stye or chalazion are fairly common and are suppurative infections of the glands of the lid (**207**). Infections of the entire lid are usually unilateral, and occur anterior to the orbital septum (**207**). While pain, swelling, and erythema occur, movement of the eye is usually normal and pain free, distinguishing this entity from orbital cellulitis. Dacrocystis is infection of the lacrymal gland, and canaliculitis is infection of the nasolacrymal duct (**212**). While common pathogens such as pneumococcus and group A streptococcus are usually responsible for acute infections, chronic infections may be caused by *Actinomyces israelii*, an actinomycete. The chronic inflammation that occurs in the duct produces a nodule, consisting of an outer layer of fibrous tissue, enclosing a purulent collection of neutrophils, which themselves surround several 'sulphur granules'. These granules contain conglomerations of bacteria, and their presence in an excised nodule is diagnostic of this condition.

Diagnosis

The various causes of conjunctivitis may be differentiated clinically (**213**). Careful collection of discharge from the conjunctival fornices of each eye must be done. A charcoal transport swab, moistened with sterile saline, can be used. For chlamydia the swab should be placed in chlamydia transport medium. Swabs for virus isolation must be placed in viral transport medium. In complicated cases of conjunctivitis, especially in the newborn, it is wise to seek the advice of the ophthalmologist before collection of specimens.

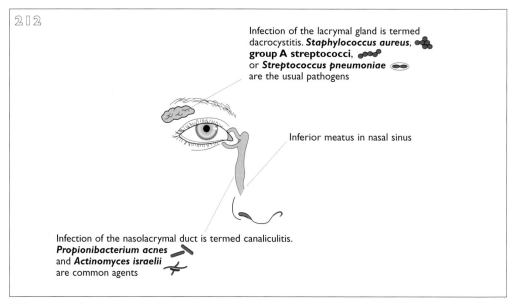

Infection of the lacrymal gland is termed dacrocystitis. **Staphylococcus aureus, group A streptococci,** or **Streptococcus pneumoniae** are the usual pathogens

Inferior meatus in nasal sinus

Infection of the nasolacrymal duct is termed canaliculitis. **Propionibacterium acnes** and **Actinomyces israelii** are common agents

212 Infections of the lacrymal gland and nasolacrymal duct.

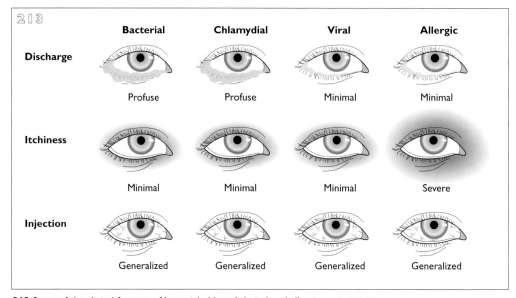

	Bacterial	Chlamydial	Viral	Allergic
Discharge	Profuse	Profuse	Minimal	Minimal
Itchiness	Minimal	Minimal	Minimal	Severe
Injection	Generalized	Generalized	Generalized	Generalized

213 Some of the clinical features of bacterial, chlamydial, viral, and allergic conjunctivitis.

For the diagnosis of keratitis it is essential to refer the patient to the ophthalmologist, as corneal scrapes need to be done, with the appropriate anaesthesia. It is important that the ophthalmologists have a close working relation with the medical microbiology laboratory in order to maximize the isolation of organisms. Corneal scrapings should be used to prepare a smear on glass slides for gram staining and to inoculate a range of culture media, including chocolate agar, and a selective agar for the isolation of fungi. In the case of contact lens wearers, corneal scrapes should be inoculated onto nutrient agar flooded with killed 'coliform' bacteria. The amoeba acanthamoeba grows by scavenging and devouring these bacteria. Plates are examined under an inverted microscope for the presence of the amoebae and their characteristic cysts.

It is possible to differentiate preseptal from orbital cellulitis on clinical grounds, for in the latter situation there is proptosis of the eye and movement is painful (**214a, b**). In endophthalmitis, fluid needs to be sent promptly to the laboratory for full microbiological investigation. In all cases of suspected endophthalmitis, orbital cellulitis and cavernous sinus thrombosis, blood cultures must be collected.

Treatment
Conjunctivitis
In most instances topical eye drops or ointment can be used to treat acute bacterial conjunctivitis. In the United Kingdom chloramphenicol is widely used; it has broad-spectrum activity and is useful for most of the common bacteria considered in **208**, with the exception of pseudomonas. The opinion that chloramphenicol should be avoided because of the risk of aplastic anaemia is not considered to be well founded. Aminoglycosides are also useful and have activity against pseudomonas. Quinolones such as ciprofloxacin and ofloxacin, and tetracyclines are also used. It is important to remember that the aminoglycosides and quinolones may have equivocal activity against streptococci, although with topical application the concentration of these agents is probably high enough to be effective. In ophthalmology departments, topical cefuroxime and gentamicin are used as these cover most of the common bacterial pathogens. Gonococcal conjunctivitis should be treated with systemic antibiotics and ceftriaxone is useful here. Regular saline washes of the eye are used to remove purulent exudate.

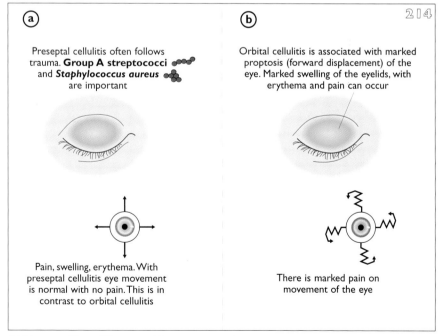

214 It is possible to differentiate (**a**) preseptal from (**b**) orbital cellulitis.

Keratitis

The agents discussed above are used here as well. Herpetic and fungal keratitis can be treated with preparations of aciclovir and amphotericin B respectively; the ophthalmologist must be consulted.

Endophthalmitis

For post-operative infections, intravitreal injection of a glycopeptide and an aminoglycoside is appropriate for most of the bacteria under consideration. In the setting of trauma, the organism that is isolated will influence the regime that is continued, but it is considered prudent to include clindamycin initially to ensure cover for *Bacillus cereus*. Penetration of antibiotics into the vitreous humour from the blood is variable. Metronidazole, RIF, chloramphenicol, co-trimoxazole, and the quinolones may achieve useful levels, but their use in the setting of endophthalmitis depends on the preference of individual ophthalmologists. In this severe infection it is not unreasonable to consider both systemic and topical agents.

Orbital cellulitis and cavernous sinus thrombosis

Antibiotics used for treating a brain abscess are useful here, and a combination of benzylpenicillin, cefotaxime and metronidazole is appropriate. Cefotaxime or ceftriaxone with clindamycin is another option. The good oral bio-availability of clindamycin and the 'once daily' intravenous regime of ceftriaxone makes this a useful combination to use in an outpatient setting for orbital cellulitis. At least 2 weeks of treatment should be considered.

Dacrocystitis and canaliculitis

Topical agents that cover the common organisms are reasonable. In the setting of actinomyces, the sulphur granule may have to be excised.

Public health issues

An important public health issue is that eye preparations should be sterile when used. In most cases eye drops are for multiple use over a number of days by the same patient, but even here it is important that the drops are not contaminated. Eye drops should not be stored longer than a few weeks after they have been opened for use. In the hospital setting, individual containers must be used for each patient, and it is prudent that these are discarded and replaced after 1 week. In outpatient and emergency ophthalmology departments, single use drops should be used. Wearers of contact lenses should be advised that cleaning must be done with fresh cleaning solutions in order to prevent contamination with acanthamoeba.

The main public health issue relating to the eye is in the underdeveloped areas of the world where onchocerciasis and trachoma are endemic. It is the provision of correct sanitation, water supplies, and elimination of vectors, combined with effective diagnostic and treatment facilities that need to be in place to combat these devastating infections.

Comment

A useful recent review is cited below:

Leibowitz HM (2000). The red eye. *New England Journal of Medicine* **343**: 345–51.

11 Infections of the Urinary Tract

Introduction

It is likely that a few bacteria enter the bladder on occasion and are flushed out at micturition. Urine should thus be regarded as sterile and hence the presence of bacteria (bacteriuria) and pus cells (pyuria) is indicative of an infective process in the renal tract.

The prevalence of UTI in various age groups is shown in **215**. In the first 3 months of life, UTI is more common in males, and can be due to structural abnormalities such as posterior urethral valves. After this period in the pre-school group of children, UTI is more common in females; infection in males is usually due to a significant structural abnormality of the renal tract. In pre-school girls, reflux of urine from the bladder into the ureters can occur. If this is associated with bacteriuria, organisms can reach the developing kidneys. Repeated infections and subsequent renal scarring can give rise to chronic renal failure.

In adults below the age of 50 years or so, UTI is rare in males, but the prevalence in females can be up to 3%. For this group there is a strong relationship between sexual activity and UTI. In the older male and female, physiological and anatomical changes of ageing predispose to chronic, often asymptomatic, bacteriuria. Some regard this as a normal consequence of the ageing process.

In the hospital setting, UTI is an important issue as it is the most common type of hospital acquired infection. Many hospital patients will have indwelling urinary catheters inserted for varying periods of time. It is reasonable to assume that any patient who has had a catheter *in situ* for 1 week or more is likely to have a chronic bacteriuria. This will only resolve when the catheter is removed.

The relevant anatomy and physiology of the urinary tract is shown in **216a**, and the routes that organisms take are indicated (**216b**). Cystitis, the most common condition, is an infection in the bladder. Bacteria can ascend the ureter

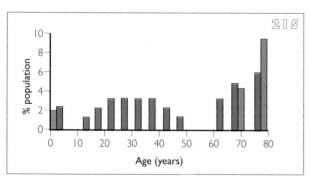

215 The prevalence of urinary tract infection in females (purple) and males (green) according to age.

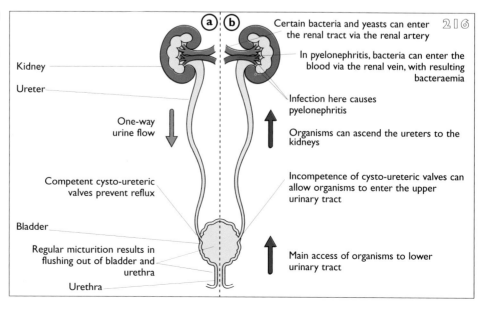

216 The renal tract. (**a**) Normal structure and physiology maintain a sterile tract. (**b**) Bacteria can enter the renal tract by the urethra or blood.

Kidney

Ureter

One-way urine flow

Competent cysto-ureteric valves prevent reflux

Bladder

Regular micturition results in flushing out of bladder and urethra

Urethra

Certain bacteria and yeasts can enter the renal tract via the renal artery

In pyelonephritis, bacteria can enter the blood via the renal vein, with resulting bacteraemia

Infection here causes pyelonephritis

Organisms can ascend the ureters to the kidneys

Incompetence of cysto-ureteric valves can allow organisms to enter the upper urinary tract

Main access of organisms to lower urinary tract

and initiate infection in the renal pelvis and kidney, which is termed pyelonephritis; from there they can enter the blood. Bacteria, including *Mycobacterium tuberculosis* and *Salmonella typhi*, as well as the candida yeasts, can enter the renal tract from the blood.

Organisms

A list of the more common organisms that cause UTI and prostatitis is shown in **217**. The 'coliforms', and *Escherichia coli* in particular, are the most common bacteria in the community. In the hospital setting, more resistant 'coliforms' such as enterobacter and citrobacter, pseudomonas, enterococci, and MRSA assume importance. Yeasts should also be considered in the catheterized patient.

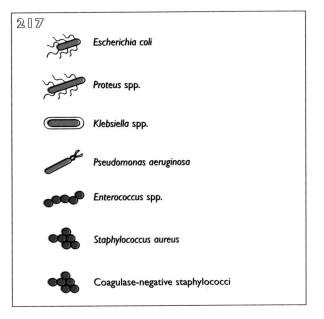

Escherichia coli

Proteus spp.

Klebsiella spp.

Pseudomonas aeruginosa

Enterococcus spp.

Staphylococcus aureus

Coagulase-negative staphylococci

217 Some of the bacteria that commonly cause urinary tract infection.

Pathogenesis

There are a number of important defences that help prevent UTI. As stated above, small numbers of bacteria are likely to ascend the urethra and enter the bladder. Regular flushing out of the bladder at micturition will remove these bacteria. This defence is aided at the microanatomical level. The bladder epithelium has a surface mucopolysaccharide which prevents small numbers of bacteria adhering to the bladder wall, thus increasing the likelihood of the bacteria being flushed out at micturition (**218**). In addition, wide variations in urine osmolarity and pH, along with the high urea concentration, can inhibit the growth of bacteria.

Normal and abnormal anatomy is central in understanding the pathogenesis of UTI. The difference between the relevant anatomies of the sexes is obvious (**219**). The male is protected by the length of the urethra and the fact that the urethral meatus opens onto the glans of the penis. The shorter urethra in the female means that bacteria have less distance to travel to reach the bladder. In addition, the urethral meatus opens into the moist introitus, which is colonized by bacteria that have the potential to cause cystitis. It is clear that sexual intercourse and the physical manipulation of the female anatomy around the urethra is likely to increase the chance of bacteria entering the bladder in significant numbers.

A model pump system where complete emptying flushes out all the bacteria present is shown in **220a**. In the setting of incomplete emptying (**220b**), a few bacteria remain and their numbers then increase. Any process which interferes with complete emptying of the bladder will have the same result. Examples include posterior urethral valves in the newborn male or prostatic enlargement in the older male.

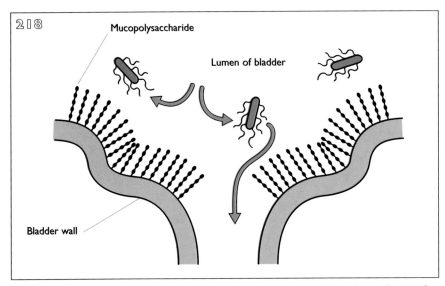

Mucopolysaccharide

Lumen of bladder

Bladder wall

218 The bladder wall is covered with a surface mucopolysaccharide that inhibits the attachment of bacteria via their adhesins.

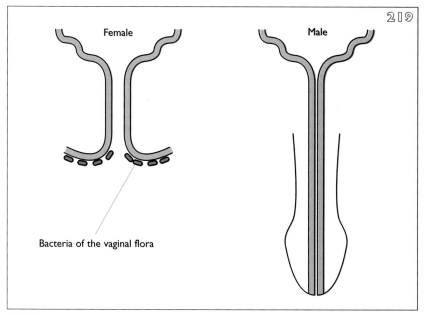

219 The shorter urethra is a predisposing factor for urinary tract infection in the female.

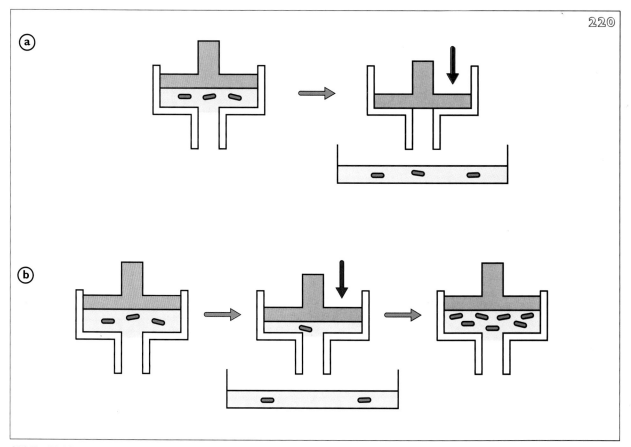

220 The bladder can be likened to a pump. (**a**) Complete emptying will flush out all the bacteria. (**b**) Incomplete emptying will leave bacteria in the residual fluid where they will reproduce.

The bladder is innervated by both sympathetic and parasympathetic nerves, which control the bladder and sphincters. Compromise of nerve function following injury to the spinal cord or in diabetes can affect bladder emptying. Some examples of physiological and anatomical abnormalities that predispose to infection are shown in **221**.

In a patient with recurrent UTI, anatomical abnormalities need to be identified and treated. This is of particular relevance in the young child, where recurrent infection is likely to cause irreversible damage to the developing kidneys. As discussed above, urethral catheters compromise the structural and physiological barriers of the urethra and bladder. Bacteria and yeasts can ascend the outside or the lumen of the catheter to reach the bladder (**222**).

An important consideration in UTI is the pathogenic properties of the bacteria themselves. This is highlighted by certain uropathogenic strains of *Escherichia coli* that are able to colonize the periurethral area of the female, ascend the urethra, and attach to the wall of the bladder. Adhesins are essential here; bacteria that adhere are less likely to be flushed out of the bladder. They can set up a nidus of infection that will progress to cystitis. From here they can ascend the ureter to reach the renal pelvis and kidney (**223**). In the bladder the growing population of bacteria incites an inflammatory response, with inflow of neutrophils.

221

Normal renal pelvis

An abnormal renal pelvis obstructs normal urine outflow

Normal cysto-ureteric junction

An abnormal cysto-ureteric junction causes reflux of urine

Normal innervation to bladder sphincters

Abnormal innervation to bladder and sphincters results in incomplete bladder emptying

Normal prostate and urethra

Diseased prostate and abnormal urethra

221 Some details of the anatomy and innervation of the renal tract in preventing and predisposing to urinary tract infection.

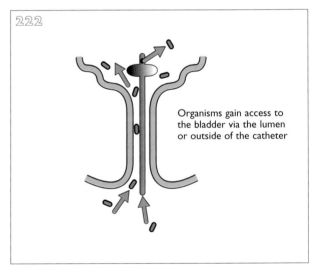

222

Organisms gain access to the bladder via the lumen or outside of the catheter

222 The insertion of a urinary catheter compromises the structural integrity of the urethra.

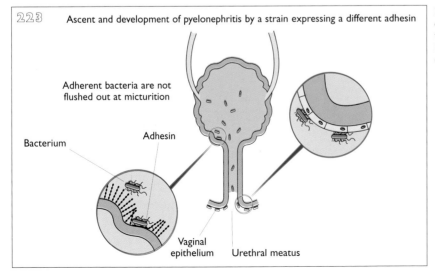

223   Ascent and development of pyelonephritis by a strain expressing a different adhesin

Adherent bacteria are not flushed out at micturition

Bacterium

Adhesin

Vaginal epithelium   Urethral meatus

223 Uropathogenic strains of *Escherichia coli* from the periurethral area can enter the bladder and attach to the wall. Expression of different adhesins allows certain bacteria to ascend to the kidney.

Bacterial toxins, as well as enzymes and other metabolites released from dead and dying neutrophils, irritate the epithelial lining of the bladder and urethra, and the classic symptoms of frequency, urgency and dysuria arise (**224**).

It is also likely that there is a genetic predisposition in females with blood group non-secretor phenotypes. These individuals express carbohydrate receptors on their vaginal epithelial cells, which are the receptors for the adhesins of uropathogenic strains of *Escherichia coli*. These bacteria colonize the periurethral area in significant numbers, from where they can ascend the urethra to the bladder.

Bacteria can reach the prostate by the urethra, lymphatics, and blood to initiate prostatitis (**225**). Instrumentation of the bladder can also introduce bacteria into the prostate. The inflamed prostate can compress the lumen of the urethra to cause obstruction, resulting in retention of urine. Prostatitis can be divided into acute or chronic disease.

On occasion, repeated specimens of urine show pus cells in the absence of any of the organisms usually associated with UTI. This sterile pyuria may be associated with chlamydial urethritis and also occurs with renal TB. A foreign body or a malignancy of the renal tract and pelvic organs are other causes of sterile pyuria.

Diagnosis

In the sexually active female, the classic symptoms of an uncomplicated UTI or cystitis are frequency, urgency, and dysuria. In other age groups these symptoms may not be elicited. Failure to thrive or poor feeding may be symptoms in the newborn. In the elderly, bedridden patient, confusion may be an indication of a UTI. In the catheterized patient with a chronic bacteriuria, fever with or without rigors can indicate that bacteria have entered the blood.

Examining a freshly collected specimen of urine by eye enables an initial assessment of a UTI. Rapid tests are also available and include urine dipsticks which can detect leucocyte esterases and nitrites, the latter being metabolic products of bacteria such as 'coliforms'. Dipsticks can be very useful to rule out a UTI; clear urine that is dipstick negative for both leucocyte esterase and nitrites means that infection is unlikely and the urine can usually be discarded. For the patient with symptoms of dysuria, urgency, and frequency whose urine is cloudy and dipstick test positive, empirical antibiotics can be prescribed and a specimen sent to the laboratory for examination. A photograph of urine after collection, and the use of dipsticks is shown in **226**.

224 In the bladder, the attached bacteria multiply and invoke an inflammatory response.

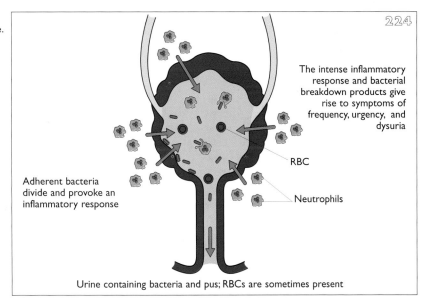

224

The intense inflammatory response and bacterial breakdown products give rise to symptoms of frequency, urgency, and dysuria

RBC

Neutrophils

Adherent bacteria divide and provoke an inflammatory response

Urine containing bacteria and pus; RBCs are sometimes present

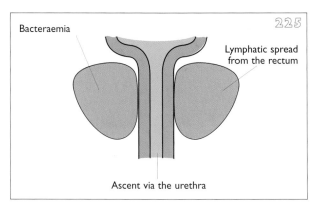

225

Bacteraemia

Lymphatic spread from the rectum

Ascent via the urethra

225 Bacteria can enter the prostate via the urethra, blood, or lymphatics.

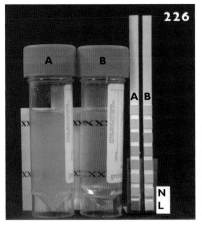

226

226 A photograph of urine specimens and dipsticks. Specimen A is cloudy and leucocyte- (L) and nitrite (N)-positive, specimen B is clear and dipstick-negative.

The usefulness of laboratory examination of urine depends on the standard of the specimen collected; a 'clean catch' urine specimen is important (**227a**). When such a specimen is obtained from an adult female with a suspected uncomplicated UTI, pus cells and a single type of bacteria should be present. In incorrectly collected specimens, vaginal epithelial cells and the bacterial flora attached to these cells will also be present. Vaginal epithelial cells are thus an indication of a contaminated specimen, which is confirmed when culture shows a mixture of bacteria (**227b**). Regular collection of urine specimens from the patient who has a long-term urinary catheter is often of doubtful use, and the practice should be discouraged. In such patients, urine should be collected for analysis only if the patient is systemically unwell, and before empirical antibiotics are prescribed.

Large numbers of urine specimens are submitted to the laboratory and semi-automated systems may be used to process the workload. An outline of a standard method of examining an individual urine specimen is shown in **228a, b**. Each specimen should be examined by low power microscopy, and the presence of WBC, RBC, and vaginal epithelial cells reported. If there are >50 WBC/μL of urine and no vaginal epithelial cells are seen, a pyuria is likely. A volume of urine is then inoculated onto selective and susceptibility testing agar. CLED is one agar that is commonly used, as it grows most of the bacteria associated with UTI and it prevents the 'swarming' by *Proteus* spp. When WBC are present in the urine, antibiotic susceptibilities are determined using the urine as the inoculum.

After overnight incubation the number of colonies is recorded and reported along with the antibiotic susceptibilities. Two examples of urine reports are shown in **229a, b**. A UTI in the female patient can usually be confirmed in the setting of pus cells, absence of vaginal epithelial cells, and a pure growth of bacteria of >10^4 cfu/mL of urine. If one or two of these parameters is not satisfied the relevance of the result needs to be reconsidered.

In the setting of pyelonephritis the patient may have the symptoms of a lower UTI as well as loin pain, fever, and rigors. Renal angle tenderness may be elicited, indicating an inflammatory process in the kidney. Blood cultures should be collected in addition to a urine specimen. In the patient who has been catheterized for longer than 7 days, a chronic bacteriuria will be present. Urine should only be collected for microbiological examination if the patient has systemic symptoms such as a fever. A change in the mental status of an elderly patient warrants a urine specimen being examined; blood culture should also be considered. The symptoms and signs of acute and chronic prostatitis are shown in **230a, b**.

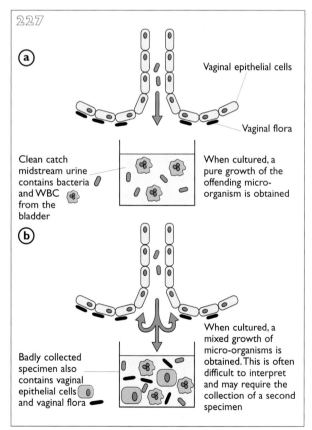

227 (a) In the female patient a 'clean catch' urine specimen will represent the contents of the bladder. **(b)** A contaminated specimen will contain vaginal epithelial cells and attached bacteria. (WBC: white blood cell.)

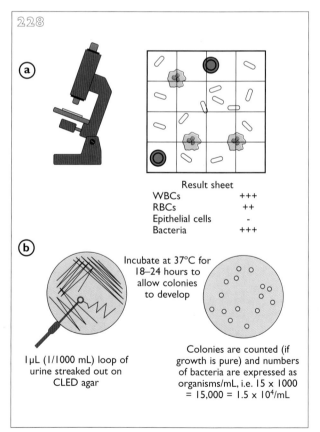

228 (a) Urine microscopy can be used to determine the presence of white blood cells (WBCs) and red blood cells (RBCs), epithelial cells, and bacteria. **(b)** A volume of urine is plated out onto a selective medium such as CLED.

When there is evidence of sterile pyuria, chlamydia infection should be promptly investigated. Where renal TB is possible, early morning urine specimens collected on 3 consecutive days should be sent to the laboratory for culture. Note that microscopy for mycobacteria is not done on these specimens, as non-pathogenic mycobacteria may be present in a specimen of urine, and thus a positive microscopy result would be meaningless.

Treatment

The common organisms and antibiotics used in the treatment of UTI infections are shown in **231**. Uncomplicated UTI in an otherwise healthy adult female patient is usually treated with a 3 day course of an oral agent. The general practitioner (GP) may prescribe an antibiotic and not send a urine specimen to the laboratory. Local antibiotic susceptibility patterns may influence the decision, and microbiology laboratories should be able to issue yearly information on the prevalence of organisms causing UTI and their susceptibility patterns.

In the community setting 'coliforms' account for about 85% of the bacteria isolated from urine specimens. Of these, at least 50% would be resistant to amoxycillin, and at least 20% resistant to trimethoprim. Amoxycillin would seldom be used empirically and with trimethoprim there may be an unacceptable failure rate. A GP may use more

a Bacteriology report			229

Name: J. Smith No.: 123456 Sex: Female DOB: 2/7/76

Diagnosis: Dysuria ?UTI Antibiotics: None Specimen: Urine

Microscopy: WBC = +++ Epithelial cells –
RBC = + Bacteria = +++

Culture: >10^4 CFU/mL coliform

Sensitive to: Cephalexin, nitrofurantoin, ciprofloxacin, co-amoxiclav
Resistant to: Ampicillin, trimethoprim

b Bacteriology report		

Name: J. Smith No.: 123456 Sex: Female DOB: 2/7/76

Diagnosis: Dysuria ?UTI Antibiotics: None Specimen: Urine

Microscopy: WBC = + Epithelial cells = +++
RBC = + Bacteria = +

Culture: Mixed growth of coliforms and enterococci
Contaminated specimen. Please send repeat specimen if clinically indicated

229 Two reports on the same patient. (**a**) Is useful and aids the management of the patient, while (**b**) is not.

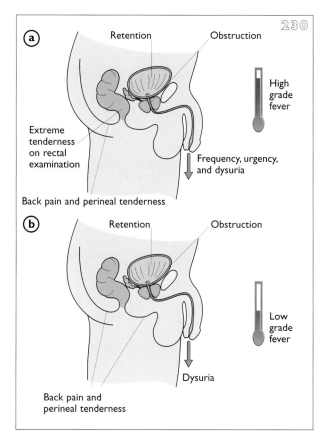

230 The symptoms and signs of (**a**) acute and (**b**) chronic prostatitis.

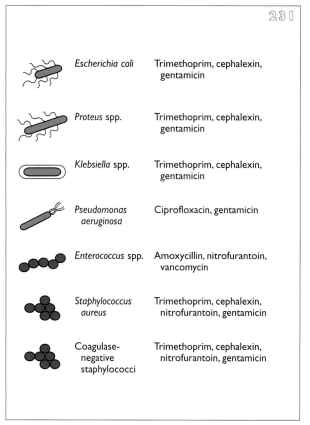

231 The common organisms that can cause urinary tract infection and antibiotics to use in treatment.

expensive agents such as cephalexin, knowing that they would be effective against over 90% of 'coliforms' isolated from community specimens. Antibiotics such as co-amoxiclav and ciprofloxacin should be reserved for cases where more resistant bacteria are isolated.

In the setting of pyelonephritis in a young adult female attending the emergency unit of a hospital, and where *Escherichia coli* is the likely organism, oral ciprofloxacin and a single pulse-dose of gentamicin is useful. If the patient improves promptly, she can be discharged home to complete a 7 day course of ciprofloxacin. The patient who is septic from a renal source needs intravenous antibiotics initially. Amoxycillin, in the patient without a penicillin allergy, and gentamicin would be a suitable empirical treatment covering both enterococci and gram-negative bacteria.

In acute prostatitis, antibiotics can penetrate the inflamed prostate tissue. In chronic prostatitis, antibiotic sensitive bacteria are isolated even after repeat courses of antibiotics. Prostatic calculi colonized with bacteria may act as foci for recurrent infection as penetration of antibiotics into the chronically infected prostate is not good. These cases may be difficult to treat, and there should be close cooperation between the physician and medical microbiologist in the management of these patients.

Public health issues

UTIs are the commonest type of hospital acquired infection. In hospitals, good standards of hygiene and infection control are essential. Urine from catheter bags should be carefully disposed of, particularly if it contains a resistant organism such as MRSA. When these resistant bacteria are involved, the patient should be nursed in a side room. Hand washing after contact with the patient must be done. Medical staff of all grades may need continual reminding of this fact.

In the sexually active female who has recurrent UTI, the association between UTI and sexual activity should be raised and the patient and her partner counselled. It may be that micturition after intercourse resolves the situation. A prophylactic antibiotic such as low dose nitrofurantoin after intercourse is another option.

Comment

The references cited below provide useful further reading and background:

Anonymous (1997). The management of urinary tract infection in children. *Drug and Therapeutic Bulletin* **35**: 65–9.

Hooton TM, Scholes D, Hughes JP et al. (1996). A prospective study of risk factors for symptomatic urinary tract infection in young women. *New England Journal of Medicine* **335**: 468–74. (Also see editorial comment on page 511.)

Hooton TM, Scholes D, Stapleton, AE et al. (2000). A prospective study of asymptomatic bacteriuria in sexually active young women. *New England Journal of Medicine* **343**: 992–7. (Also see editorial comment on pages 1037–9.)

Stamm WE, Hooton TM (1993) Management of urinary tract infections in adults. *New England Journal of Medicine* **329**: 1328–34.

12 Infections of the Genital Systems

Introduction

This chapter is primarily concerned with diseases of the female genital tract, congenital infections of the developing fetus, and perinatal infections of the newborn. A wide range of organisms is considered here, including group B streptococcus, *Listeria monocytogenes,* gonococcus, syphilis, chlamydia, rubella virus, HBV, and HIV. The three viruses are discussed here in view of their importance in congenital and perinatal infections. It should be recognized that the most common infections of the anogenital tract are caused by the human papilloma viruses (HPVs). Their importance is exemplified by the clear relationship between HPV 16 and 18 and cervical carcinoma.

Sexually transmitted diseases (STDs) such as chlamydia and gonorrhoea are well recognized, and for an individual presenting with a first episode of urethritis, the diagnosis and treatment may be straightforward. However, this person must have been infected during sexual intercourse. Sexual partners should be traced in order to identify and eliminate infections in those individuals as well. This is so important as infection can be asymptomatic, especially in females. In the case of chlamydia, it is likely that only 10% of infected individuals seek medical advice, emphasizing the difference between a sexually transmitted infection (STI) and a STD for which medical help is usually sought.

The more promiscuous a person is, the greater the chance that they will acquire at least one STI. Vaginal, anal, and oral sex need to be considered in the assessment of the patient. Gonococcus can cause urethritis, cervicitis, proctitis, and pharyngitis; pharyngeal carriage of the organism is often asymptomatic. Pelvic inflammatory disease (PID) is a complication of both gonococcal and chlamydial infection; other organisms of the vaginal flora are also involved in recurrent or chronic disease. Important complications of PID are ectopic pregnancy and infertility.

Vaginal discharges include bacterial vaginosis, often associated with the gram-negative or gram-variable bacterium *Gardnerella vaginalis,* candidiasis caused by the candida yeasts, and trichomoniasis caused by the protozoal parasite *Trichomonas vaginalis.* Trichomoniasis may be linked to sexual activity, as there is a probable relationship between this condition and the number of sexual partners. The presence of trichomonas in a specimen should prompt a search for gonococcus and chlamydia.

Pregnancy is usually a healthy state for the expectant mother, but the main concern here is the transmission of organisms to the fetus and newborn. It is for this reason that expectant mothers are screened at their first antenatal visit for immunity to rubella virus, past exposure to syphilis, and chronic carriage of HBV and HIV infection. Early identification of any of these agents enables appropriate medical management to be actioned. Infections that can be acquired by the developing fetus include the parasite *Toxoplasma gondii,* rubella virus, CMV, HSV, and syphilis, which are the basis of the 'TORCHES screen' when abnormalities are detected during pregnancy or noted after birth. As other organisms such as parvovirus B19 also cause congenital infection, the 'TORCHES screen' is a somewhat dated term.

The newborn child is at risk of infection arising from acquisition of organisms from the normal vaginal flora, for example group B streptococcus and *Escherichia coli.* Pathogens in the mother's bowel, such as listeria, can reach the fetus via a maternal bacteraemia.

Post-partum infections, endometritis and septic abortions are other important conditions to consider, as are infections arising from gynaecological procedures such as vaginal and abdominal hysterectomy.

An outline of the female genital tract and the organisms that make up the normal vaginal flora are shown in **232a, b.** Organisms can reach the uterine adnexae via the uterus and

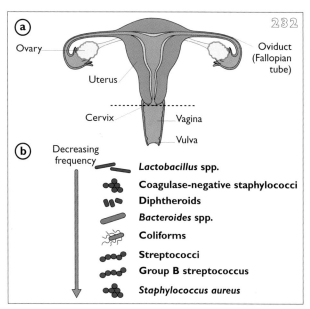

232 (a) An outline of the female genital tract. **(b)** Bacteria that make up the normal vaginal flora.

Fallopian tubes, as occurs in PID. Because of the proximity of the introitus to the anus, it is not surprising that the vaginal flora includes organisms of faecal origin. It is important to appreciate the changes in the physiology and bacterial flora of the tract in the life of the female, as shown diagrammatically in **233**. It is relevant to note that the vaginal epithelium in the pre-pubertal age is not keratinized and will support the growth of gonococcus. Any vaginal discharge in a pre-pubertal girl must be examined for gonococcus, as well as chlamydia, to rule out sexual abuse.

The normal vaginal flora also varies during the menstrual cycle, with a mixed bacterial flora in the follicular phase and lactobacilli dominating the luteal phase (**234**). In the luteal phase, lactobacilli use the glycogen in sloughed vaginal epithelial cells, with lactic acid end products being important in maintaining the acid milieu of the vagina.

Organisms

A list of the organisms considered in the various clinical settings is shown in **235**. Rubella virus, HBV, and HIV are important congenital and perinatal viral infections and are considered here. Syphilis is caused by the spirochete *Treponema pallidum*.

Pathogenesis
Sexually transmitted diseases: gonorrhoea and chlamydia
Gonorrhoea

The causative agent of gonorrhoea is *Neisseria gonorrhoeae*, a gram-negative diplococcus, which infects the columnar and cuboidal epithelia to cause cervicitis, urethritis, proctitis, and pharyngitis (**236a–e**). In the endocervix and Fallopian tubes, the organism attaches to columnar epithelial cells by adhesins and the cell wall outer membrane opa proteins. Following attachment, invasion of the epithelium and sub-epithelium occurs. The strong inflammatory response is associated with neutrophil invasion, micro-abscess formation, and pus.

Infection in the female can be asymptomatic, but in males an acute urethritis is the usual presenting symptom. Gonococcus can reach the epididymis of the male to initiate epididymitis, and the Fallopian tubes and adnexa in the female, where it is involved in PID. In the newborn, acquisition of the organism at birth can give rise to ophthalmia neonatorum.

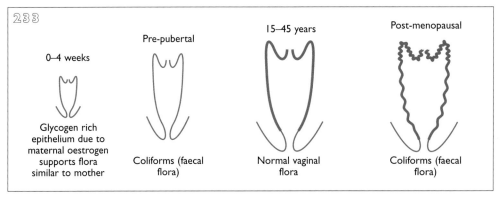

233 Changes that occur in the bacterial flora of the vagina in the various ages.

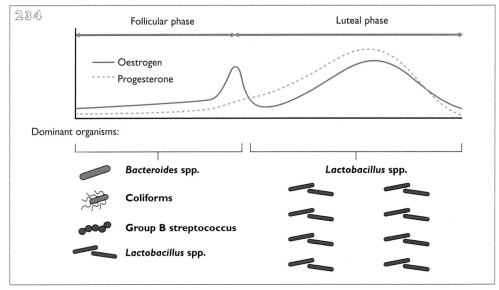

234 The menstrual cycle, with the changes that occur with the bacterial flora during the cycle.

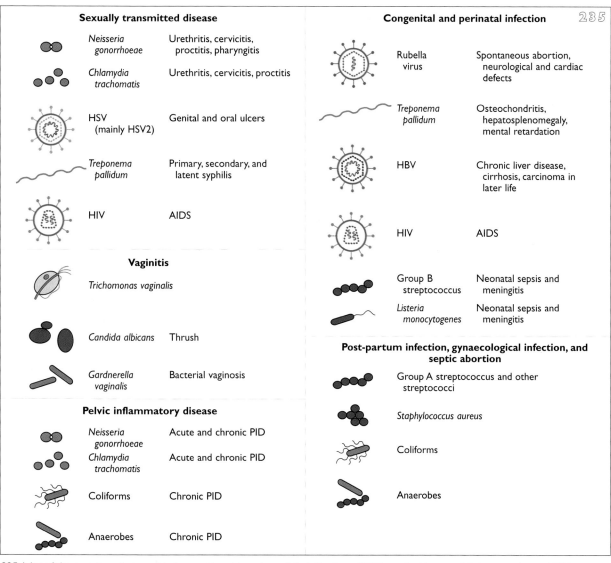

Sexually transmitted disease

	Neisseria gonorrhoeae	Urethritis, cervicitis, proctitis, pharyngitis
	Chlamydia trachomatis	Urethritis, cervicitis, proctitis
	HSV (mainly HSV2)	Genital and oral ulcers
	Treponema pallidum	Primary, secondary, and latent syphilis
	HIV	AIDS

Vaginitis

	Trichomonas vaginalis	
	Candida albicans	Thrush
	Gardnerella vaginalis	Bacterial vaginosis

Pelvic inflammatory disease

	Neisseria gonorrhoeae	Acute and chronic PID
	Chlamydia trachomatis	Acute and chronic PID
	Coliforms	Chronic PID
	Anaerobes	Chronic PID

Congenital and perinatal infection

	Rubella virus	Spontaneous abortion, neurological and cardiac defects
	Treponema pallidum	Osteochondritis, hepatosplenomegaly, mental retardation
	HBV	Chronic liver disease, cirrhosis, carcinoma in later life
	HIV	AIDS
	Group B streptococcus	Neonatal sepsis and meningitis
	Listeria monocytogenes	Neonatal sepsis and meningitis

Post-partum infection, gynaecological infection, and septic abortion

	Group A streptococcus and other streptococci
	Staphylococcus aureus
	Coliforms
	Anaerobes

235 A list of the organisms that need to be considered in various clinical situations. (AIDS: acquired immunodeficiency syndrome; HIV: human immunodeficiency virus; HSV: herpes simplex virus; PID: pelvic inflammatory disease.)

236 In gonococcal disease the organism can cause infection in the (**a**) cervix; (**b**) urethra and epididymis; (**c**) female urethra; (**d**) anus; (**e**) pharynx.

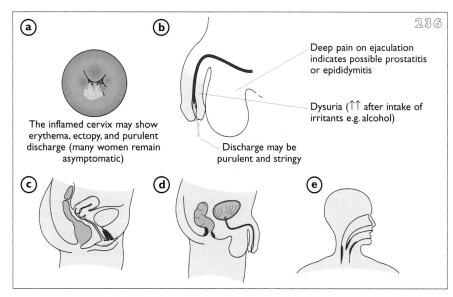

(**a**) The inflamed cervix may show erythema, ectopy, and purulent discharge (many women remain asymptomatic)

(**b**) Deep pain on ejaculation indicates possible prostatitis or epididymitis

Dysuria (↑↑ after intake of irritants e.g. alcohol)

Discharge may be purulent and stringy

Chlamydia trachomatis

Chlamydia are obligate intracellular bacteria. There are several serological groups or serovars, with the A, B and C serovars associated with ocular trachoma and the D to K serovars associated with inclusion conjunctivitis (including ophthalmia neonatorum) and urogenital disease. Chlamydia causes urethritis, proctitis, and epididymitis in the male, urethritis and cervicitis in the female, and ophthalmia neonatorum in the newborn.

Chlamydia have a complex life cycle within infected epithelial cells. Following entry into cells, the elementary body converts to a reticulate body, the reproductive form of the organism. Reproduction occurs in an endosome, a membrane limited structure within the infected cell. Reticulate bodies produce the elementary bodies that are then released as the extracellular infective form of the organism (237).

Pelvic inflammatory disease

Acute PID arises following ascent of gonococcus and chlamydia through the uterine cavity to the Fallopian tubes and adnexae (238a–c). Both subclinical and chronic disease can then occur, where bacteria of the vaginal flora are also involved. Inflammation and fibrosis damage the Fallopian tubes, obstructing the normal movement of ova

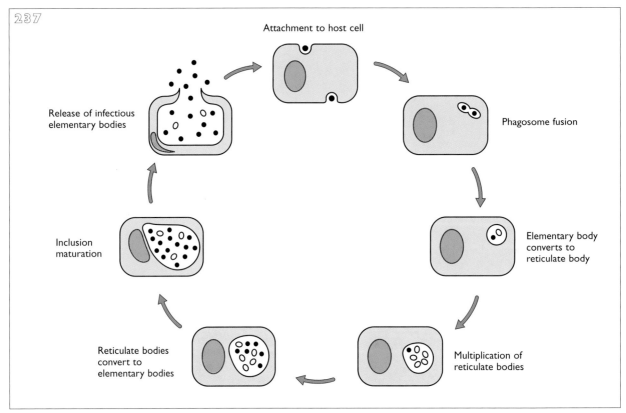

237 The life cycle of chlamydia. (●: Elementary body; ○: reticulate body.)

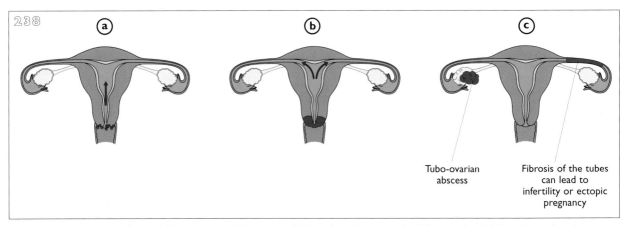

238 In pelvic inflammatory disease (**a**) bacteria ascend the uterus; (**b**) from here they enter the Fallopian tubes. (**c**) Infection in the tubes results in fibrosis and a tubo-ovarian abscess can also develop.

to the uterus. If a fertilized ovum implants in the tube, an ectopic pregnancy results, which is a gynaecological emergency. When both tubes are affected, infertility can arise. A pelvic abscess is also a complication of PID, and when on the right side, this or an ectopic pregnancy need to be differentiated from disease of the appendix.

Vaginitis

Vaginal discharges are associated with *Gardnerella vaginalis*, *Candida albicans* and other candida yeasts, and *Trichomonas vaginalis*.

Candida infections are associated with factors that change the normal flora and physiology of the vagina. Broad-spectrum antibiotics alter the vaginal flora, allowing yeasts to overgrow. The oral contraceptive is another predisposing factor, and by increasing glycogen stores in vaginal epithelial cells it enables candida to outgrow the lactobacilli. In addition, oestrogen may induce candida receptors on the surface of vaginal epithelial cells.

Gardnerella vaginalis is an organism associated with bacterial vaginosis, which is a polymicrobial condition. In addition to gardnerella, *Mycoplasma hominis* and anaerobes such as mobiluncus are involved. It is probable that these organisms have the ability to overwhelm the lactobacillus population of the vagina, with the resulting inflammatory response producing the discharge. Gardnerella is a gram-negative or gram-variable bacillus and can be detected on gram stained preparations adherent in large numbers to vaginal epithelial cells, termed 'clue' cells. Gardnerella also produces a β-haemolysin, which lyses human red blood cells. Although the role of this haemolysin is unclear, it may give gardnerella an advantage over the normal flora for available iron in the vagina, as iron is an essential factor for bacterial growth.

Growth of trichomonas is optimal in a less acidic environment, and explains the tendency for symptoms to exacerbate in progesterone-dominant states such as pregnancy and menstruation. A purulent foul-smelling frothy discharge may be present in up to half of infected individuals.

Congenital infections
Rubella

Rubella virus is a member of the Flaviviridae family. The genome of these viruses consists of single-stranded RNA, enclosed in a protein capsid. Flaviviruses also have an outer lipid envelope obtained when the virus buds through the cytoplasmic membrane of the host cell. In children and occasionally adults, rubella virus usually causes a mild febrile illness with a rash. If, however, a primary infection occurs during the first trimester of pregnancy, the effects on the fetus can be devastating. Crossing the placenta during a maternal viraemia, the virus invades a wide range of fetal tissues, affecting cell growth and organ development. A placental vasculitis compromises the blood supply to the fetus. The results of infection range from spontaneous abortion to significant congenital defects, which include microcephaly, mental retardation, cataracts, and congenital heart defects. In the first 2 months the chance of a fetus being affected ranges from 60–90%, falling to 10% by the fourth month of gestation.

Syphilis

Syphilis is a STD, with primary disease arising after sexual exposure. A painless ulcer arises at the site of inoculation. The organism then invades the blood and is distributed widely, manifesting as a rash some weeks later as secondary syphilis. At this stage, lesions on the skin and mucous membranes are teeming with organisms. The infection then enters a latent phase where symptoms and signs of active disease are absent. However, during the first 4 years or so of latent disease, relapses to the infectious state can occur. The subsequent latent phase may progress to tertiary syphilis manifesting as neurosyphilis or cardiac syphilis.

Congenital infection is most likely to occur in a pregnant woman who is in the early years of infection. Transplacental transfer of the organism is uncommon in the first 4 months of gestation. While abortion may occur, osteochondritis, hepatosplenomegaly, rash, and nasal snuffles are characteristics features in the affected newborn.

Perinatal infections
Hepatitis B virus

HBV is a DNA-containing virus, whose main target cell is the liver hepatocyte. As with most DNA viruses, HBV replicates in the nucleus of the infected cell. The viral DNA is surrounded by a core protein (cAg), and exterior to this is a lipid membrane containing the surface antigen (sAg). The majority of individuals infected with HBV become immune, producing antibodies (cAb) to the cAg, indicating past infection, and antibodies (sAb) to the sAg, which are protective.

Many DNA viruses have the ability to cause chronic infections, and in the case of HBV, chronic infection occurs in about 10% of infected individuals, although in Africa and the Far East the rates are higher. Chronic carriage is identified by serological tests, which show the individual to be cAb-positive and sAg-positive; carriers can be further divided into those who are eAg-positive or negative. The presence of this antigen is an indication of active viral replication in the liver, classing the person as 'high-risk'. Antibodies to e antigen (eAb) indicate a low-risk carrier. High-risk carriers are thus cAb+/sAg+/eAg+/eAb-, while low risk carriers are cAb+/sAg+/eAg-/eAb+.

Congenital transmission is uncommon, with most events occurring in the perinatal period. There are significant differences in the transmission rate when low- and high-risk mothers are compared. Only 5–10% of offspring become infected when the mother is low-risk, whereas 90–100% are infected if the mother is high-risk. Breastfeeding carries a low risk of transmission.

Human immunodeficiency virus

HIV is a retrovirus. After entering a cell, such as the T4 cell, the RNA genome is copied into DNA and a double-stranded form then integrates into the host chromosomal DNA as a provirus. New copies of the viral RNA are produced by transcription. HIV infection is a chronic infection, and in the natural course of the disease the viral load in the blood is highest in early and late (AIDS) stages of infection.

Less than 20% of all transmission events from HIV-positive mothers occur during gestation; the remaining

80% or so occur in the perinatal period. There is about a 1 in 3 chance of the virus passing from an HIV-positive mother to the newborn and initiating an infection. In contrast to HBV, there is an additional and significant risk of transmission of HIV with breastfeeding.

Group B streptococcus
This organism is a member of the normal vaginal flora in up to 40% of adult females. A number of factors determine the likelihood of invasive disease in the newborn, including preterm labour, prolonged rupture of membranes, multiple births, and maternal amnionitis. The bacteria invade the blood of the neonate via the mucous membranes to cause sepsis and meningitis. Preterm infants are thought to be at risk because they are likely to have lower levels of protective maternal IgG antibodies and their neutrophil reserves are low. Early disease occurs within 5 days of delivery. Late disease, from 1–4 weeks after delivery, is probably due to organisms being acquired from the hands of health care workers.

Listeria monocytogenes
This small gram-positive motile organism is associated with unpasteurized dairy products and other foods. Asymptomatic stool carriage probably occurs in at least 1% of the population. Bacteraemia is more common in pregnancy, especially in the third trimester. Listeria probably invades the blood from the bowel of the pregnant woman and from an occult bacteraemia it crosses the placenta to initiate infection in the fetus and the amniotic fluid.

Post-partum infections, septic abortions and gynaecological infections
In post-partum infections and septic abortions, organisms of the vaginal or bowel flora are important. Group A streptococcus and clostridia should always be considered as well. Damage to the myometrium, retained products of conception, and in the case of a septic abortion, uterine perforation, enable organisms to establish a focus of infection (**239a**). Caesarean section wounds may also be a focus of infection, and in the case of group A streptococcus, necrotizing fasciitis and TSS can occur. In hysterectomy operations, vaginal organisms may establish infections such as cuff cellulitis, cuff abscess, or pelvic abscess (**239b**), despite the use of prophylactic antibiotics. Obesity, diabetes, and difficult operations predispose to this.

Diagnosis
Sexually transmitted diseases: gonorrhoea and chlamydia
Gonococcus and chlamydia are the two infections routinely screened for at genito-urinary medicine (GUM) clinics. While dual infections are relatively common, patients with gonococcal urethritis (GCU) are more likely to be symptomatic than those with non-gonococcal urethritis (NGU), and males are more likely to be symptomatic than females. It is thus important that contacts of the index case are traced and screened.

Using the appropriate counselling and care before and during examination of the patient, specimens are collected using separate swabs for both gonococcus and chlamydia (**240**). (See also **55**.) As with any test, the quality of the specimen is important, particularly with an intracellular organism such as chlamydia. With the female patient it is important to remove any pus from the cervical os, so that good quality endocervical material can be collected. GUM clinics usually have microbiology technical support on site, so that microscopy can be done promptly on specimens and the result used to manage the patient. The presence of gram-negative diplococci within neutrophils may be considered diagnostic of gonococcus, particularly in a specimen from a male who presents with urethritis (**241**). In order to isolate the labile gonococcus, the swab is inoculated promptly onto selective agar plates containing vancomycin, nystatin, and trimethoprim, which inhibit the normal flora and allow the gonococcus to grow. After incubation at 37°C in an atmosphere of 5% CO_2, suspected gonococci are confirmed by gram stain, a positive oxidase test, and by rapid serological or biochemical tests. Susceptibility of the organism to penicillin, ciprofloxacin, azithromycin, and tetracycline is usually determined. Isolates that have reduced susceptibility to, or which are resistant to penicillin, will have penicillin Etest™ and β-lactamase tests done.

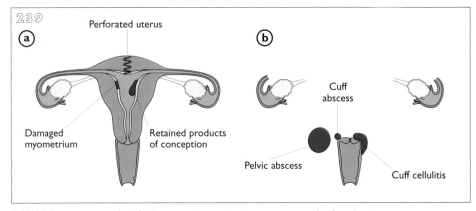

239 (a) Some reasons why infection may arise post-partum or as a result of an abortion.
(b) Some types of infection that may arise following a hysterectomy.

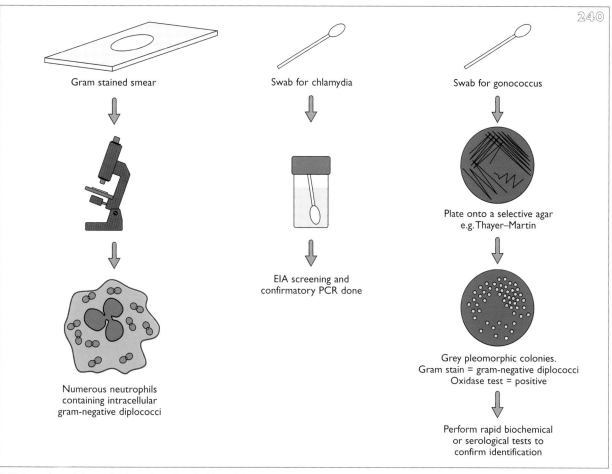

240 An outline of the methods used to identify chlamydial and gonococcal infections. (EIA: enzyme immunoassay; PCR: polymerase chain reaction.)

241 Photomicrograph of the gram stain of a urethral discharge from a male patient. Numerous gram-negative diplococci and neutrophils are seen; this patient has gonorrhoea.

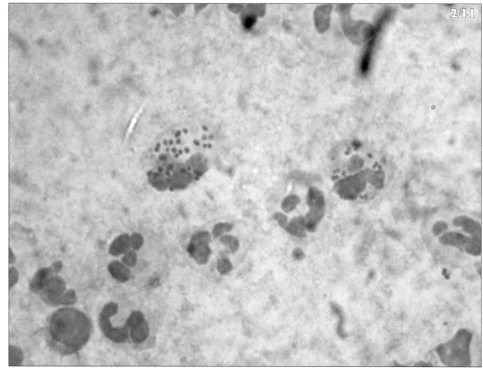

The chlamydia swab is placed in chlamydia transport medium, which can then be examined in the laboratory by a serological test such an EIA. Positive test results should be confirmed by a nucleic acid amplification test (NAAT) such as the PCR. Urine specimens can also be collected from the male patient and examined by a NAAT. Increasing use of NAAT as the single test for chlamydia is likely in coming years.

Vaginitis

The patient with a vaginal discharge should have a vaginal examination to determine the extent of the discharge and so that endocervical swabs can also be taken for the examination of gonococcus and chlamydia. Both wet films and gram stains should be examined by microscopy. Trichomonas and yeasts can readily be identified. With bacterial vaginosis, clue cells may be seen. The laboratory analysis of a vaginal discharge is shown in **242**. (See also **55**.) When a swab is taken by a GP or on the ward, a charcoal transport swab rather than a dry swab must be used, as the labile trichomonas and gonococcus should be given every opportunity to survive the trip to the laboratory. A photograph of a clue cell is shown in **243**.

Pelvic inflammatory disease

In most circumstances the diagnosis of PID is based on the clinical evidence. The patient may have a cervical discharge and internal examination shows cervical motion tenderness and a palpable pelvic mass; fever, raised WBC count, CRP, and ESR are also relevant. It is appropriate to collect endocervical swabs for gonococcus and chlamydia, and in the hospital setting, blood for culture.

Congenital infections

At the first antenatal visit, blood is collected and screened by EIA for rubella, treponemal, and HIV antibodies, as well as for HBV surface antigen. Expectant mothers should be rubella IgG-positive, indicating immunity, but treponemal and HIV antibody-negative, indicating that there is no previous exposure to these organisms. A HBV sAg negative result is used to rule out chronic infection. A report issued where further action is usually not needed is shown in **244**.

Rubella

The absence of rubella antibodies means that the woman is susceptible to rubella infection, and requires vaccination after the baby is born. As rubella vaccine is a live vaccine,

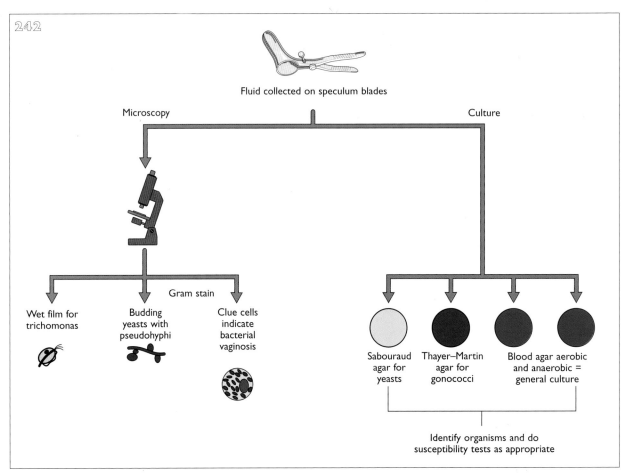

242 An outline of the methods used to investigate a vaginal discharge.

it should not be used in pregnancy. The patient should be advised about the risks of exposure to a case of rubella, particularly in the first trimester. If this occurred, she should have rubella IgM levels checked as soon as possible after the exposure and 28 days later, or 7 days after the appearance of a rubella-like rash. The appearance of IgM antibodies would indicate infection. The patient should be fully counselled by the obstetrician, who would take advice from a consultant medical virologist.

Syphilis

If the treponemal EIA is positive, further tests are performed to confirm the result and to determine if there is current active disease or latent infection. There are organism-specific tests such as the treponemal IgM and *Treponema pallidum* haemagglutination assay (TPHA) or the particle agglutination assay (TPPA). In addition, a non-treponemal test is also done. The usual test here is the Venereal Diseases Reference Laboratory (VDRL), which determines the presence of antibodies to cardiolipin. As syphilis is a vasculitic disease, raised VDRL antibodies can indicate active infection.

A positive VDRL result needs to take into account the fact that the VDRL is also raised by other conditions such as liver disease and pregnancy itself, but the titre here is usually <1/8. A VDRL value of >1/8 in the setting of positive specific treponemal tests indicates active infection. The level of antibodies at stages of the disease is shown in **245**. The person whose blood is taken at point A has both raised treponemal and VDRL antibodies and active disease is likely. The specimen taken at point B, where VDRL titres are low, is in the stage of latent infection. Transmission of the organism to the fetus is most likely to occur when the mother is in the early years of infection. However, new cases identified at antenatal screening that have the serological characteristics of latent infection should be considered for treatment and referred to the GUM clinic. The healthy newborn whose mother is treponemal antibody-positive can be monitored for loss of passively acquired maternal IgG antibodies in the first few months following delivery.

Hepatitis B virus

When the mother is identified as a HBV carrier, being sAg-positive, the eAg and eAb markers are also determined. The individual who is eAg-positive and eAb-negative is 'high risk', whereas the result of eAg-negative and eAb-positive would be 'low risk'.

Human immunodeficiency virus

The identification of HIV antibodies in pregnancy will necessitate further investigation of the mother, the staging of her infection, determination of the HIV viral load, and institution of antiviral chemotherapy. After birth, the infant needs to be monitored for the presence of HIV infection. This involves screening for the p24 viral core antigen, as well as the virus genome in the form of both RNA and DNA provirus.

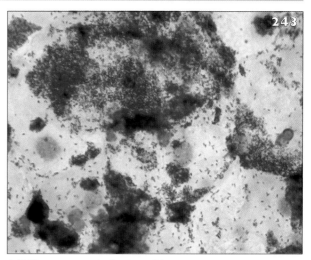

243 Photomicrograph of a clue cell from a patient with bacterial vaginosis.

Virology report	244

Name: J. Smith	No.: 123456	Sex: Female	DOB: 2/2/76

Diagnosis: Pregnant   Specimen: Blood

Rubella antibodies:	DETECTED
Treponema pallidum antibodies:	NOT detected
HIV antibodies:	NOT detected
Hepatitis B virus surface antigen:	NOT detected

244 Based on a single blood test, the antenatal screening result shows that there is usually no risk to the fetus of rubella, syphilis, hepatitis B virus, or human immunodeficiency virus infection.

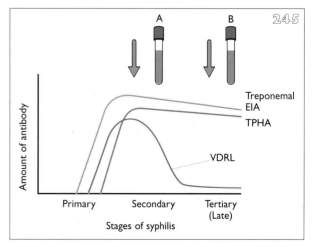

245 The time course in the appearance of antibodies to syphilis in both treponemal and non-treponemal tests. A specimen taken at point A is likely to indicate active disease, whereas the specimen taken at point B is likely to indicate latent disease. (EIA: enzyme immunoassay; TPHA: *Treponema pallidum* haemagglutination; VDRL: Venereal Disease Reference Laboratory.)

Group B streptococcus and listeria

In the case of suspected infection with group B strepto-coccus or listeria, genital swabs, specimens of amniotic fluid, and blood cultures can be collected. The newborn should have nose, ear, and perineal swabs, and blood culture collected.

Treatment

The treatment options for various conditions are shown in **246**. Tetracyclines such as doxycycline are useful monotherapy for both gonococcus and chlamydia where gonococcal isolates are routinely sensitive to the agent. Tetracyclines must not be used in pregnancy, as they affect the development of teeth in the fetus. Combined with metronidazole, doxycycline is also useful for treating PID.

In chronic PID, anaerobes, streptococci and coliforms need to be considered. If there is no response to doxycycline and metronidazole, clindamycin and ciprofloxacin are a useful oral combination to consider. In the hospital setting, gentamicin can be used instead of ciprofloxacin.

Invasive disease by listeria and group B streptococcus in the newborn can be treated with a combination of benzylpenicillin (or amoxycillin) and gentamicin. In puerperal sepsis, benzylpenicillin, gentamicin, and metro-nidazole are an acceptable broad-spectrum combination. Where group A streptococcus is identified in puerperal sepsis, benzylpenicillin and clindamycin are the combin-ation of choice. In the setting of necrotizing fasciitis associated with a caesarean section wound, urgent surgical review of the patient must be made.

In order to protect the newborn whose mother has chronic HBV infection, the first of four doses of the HBV vaccine is given within 48 hours of birth. In addition to vaccine, offspring of high-risk mothers are also given HBV immune globulin as protective passive immunity. The vast majority of children who have this intervention are protected. With HIV in pregnancy, antiviral therapy in the mother should reduce the viral load and thus the chance of transmission to the newborn. Caesarian section and the use of zidovudine for the first 6 weeks of life in the child significantly reduce the likelihood of disease developing. Transmission rates fall from one in three with no intervention to less than one in 20 with intervention.

Public health issues

The diagnosis and treatment of infections associated with sexual activity constitute a significant part of health care expenditure. GUM clinics enable individuals to be investigated with the appropriate confidentiality. Codes are used to preserve anonymity, so that outside the clinic test requests and results do not reveal the identity of the individual. HIV- and HBV-positive mothers must be managed with the correct confidential procedures as well, and this requires the correct lines of communication from the laboratory to all health care workers involved in the management of the mother and her child, as well as family and other social contacts.

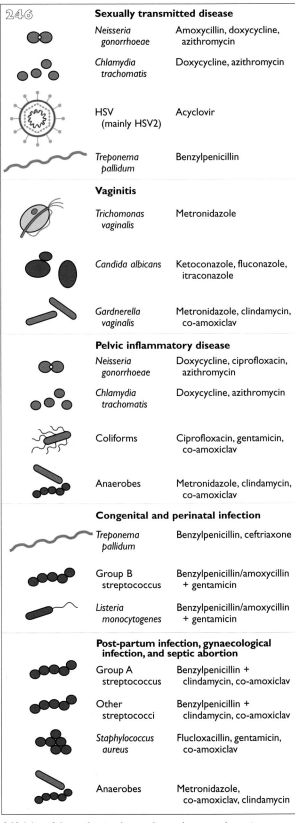

246

Sexually transmitted disease	
Neisseria gonorrhoeae	Amoxycillin, doxycycline, azithromycin
Chlamydia trachomatis	Doxycycline, azithromycin
HSV (mainly HSV2)	Acyclovir
Treponema pallidum	Benzylpenicillin
Vaginitis	
Trichomonas vaginalis	Metronidazole
Candida albicans	Ketoconazole, fluconazole, itraconazole
Gardnerella vaginalis	Metronidazole, clindamycin, co-amoxiclav
Pelvic inflammatory disease	
Neisseria gonorrhoeae	Doxycycline, ciprofloxacin, azithromycin
Chlamydia trachomatis	Doxycycline, azithromycin
Coliforms	Ciprofloxacin, gentamicin, co-amoxiclav
Anaerobes	Metronidazole, clindamycin, co-amoxiclav
Congenital and perinatal infection	
Treponema pallidum	Benzylpenicillin, ceftriaxone
Group B streptococcus	Benzylpenicillin/amoxycillin + gentamicin
Listeria monocytogenes	Benzylpenicillin/amoxycillin + gentamicin
Post-partum infection, gynaecological infection, and septic abortion	
Group A streptococcus	Benzylpenicillin + clindamycin, co-amoxiclav
Other streptococci	Benzylpenicillin + clindamycin, co-amoxiclav
Staphylococcus aureus	Flucloxacillin, gentamicin, co-amoxiclav
Anaerobes	Metronidazole, co-amoxiclav, clindamycin

246 A list of the antibiotics that can be used to treat the various infections considered in this chapter. (HSV: herpes simplex virus.)

Screening in the community for chlamydia should be a priority, as asymptomatic infection is common, and causes PID and infertility. For this reason, programs need to be introduced in communities for individuals in higher risk categories to be screened. It has been shown that nucleic acid tests such PCR done on urine specimens provide a useful non-invasive method for this purpose. The importance of screening, vaccination, and other procedures to prevent the transmission of infections to the fetus and newborn has to be emphasized.

Comment

Invasive disease by group B streptococcus is a well recognized entity in newborns. Maternal colonization is a prerequisite for infection, with other risk factors being pre-term delivery, prolonged rupture of membranes, and a multiple pregnancy.

Some useful references on this subject are listed below:

Bergeron MG, Ke D, Menard C *et al.* (2000). Rapid detection of group B streptococcus in pregnant women at delivery. *New England Journal of Medicine* 343(3): 175–9. (Also see editorial comment on pages 209–210.)

Editorial (1995). Group B streptococcus: the US controversy. *Lancet* **346**: 197–8.

Goldenberg RL, Hauth JC, Andrews WW (2000). Intrapartum infection and preterm delivery. *New England Journal of Medicine* **342**: 1500–6.

Schrag SJ, Ziwicki S, Farley MM *et al.* (2000). Group B streptococcal disease in the era of interpartum antibiotic prophylaxis. *New England Journal of Medicine* **342**: 15–20.

It is important that both the obstetricians and neonatologists have protocols for the management of group B infection in the peri-partum period, based on national guidelines. The following are a reasonable basis for such guidelines:

Women with one or more of the following:
- group B streptococcus bacteriuria in the current pregnancy;
- vaginal carriage group B streptococcus in the current pregnancy;
- a previous preterm delivery or pregnancy loss associated with group B streptococcus.

Should be treated with antibiotics if they present with:
- preterm labour (<37 weeks), with or without rupture of membranes;
- prolonged rupture of membranes;
- maternal fever in labour.

The antibiotics used are benzylpenicillin or, in the case of a penicillin allergy, clindamycin. While the streptococcus can be considered to be routinely sensitive to penicillin, resistance to erythromycin and thus clindamycin does occur. Antibiotics should usually be continued until delivery.

13 Infections of the Skin, Soft Tissues, Joints and Bone

Introduction

Infections of the skin and soft tissues include a wide range of clinical situations and organisms (**247**). Many of these infections arise following a breach of the skin, emphasizing the importance of this natural barrier. Once the skin is breached, organisms can enter the deeper soft tissue. Any surgical incision compromises the barrier, and wound infections are an important entity in hospital acquired infection. Bacteria such as *Staphylococcus aureus*, including MRSA, and group A streptococcus are important pathogens here. The bite of a dog or cat can introduce members of the oral flora of these animals such as *Pasteurella multocida* and *Eikinella corrodens*, and may result in serious local and systemic infection.

Staphylococci and streptococci are the commoner causes of infections of the joints and bone. *Haemophilus influenzae* b was a common cause of arthritis and osteomyelitis in children under 5 years. However, such invasive disease is now rare in countries where Hib vaccination is practised.

In the individual with a chronic joint infection, it is always important to consider a wider range of organisms, and mycobacteria are an example. Any patient with chronic infection of joints of the hand must be asked if they keep tropical fish. *Mycobacterium marinum* is commonly found in tropical fish tanks, and after entering a skin abrasion, it can cause an infection. The medical microbiologist needs to be informed here, as any biopsy tissue should be incubated

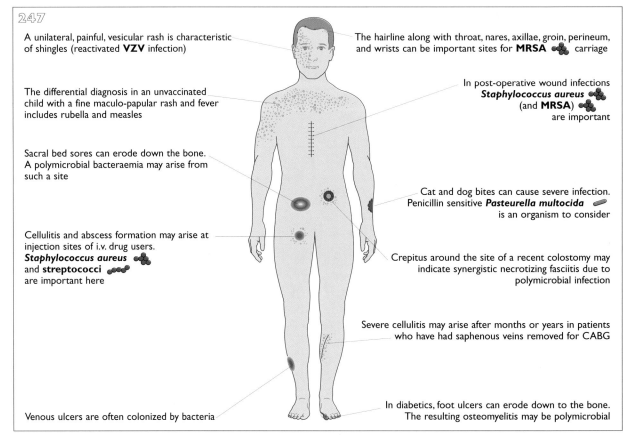

247

A unilateral, painful, vesicular rash is characteristic of shingles (reactivated **VZV** infection)

The differential diagnosis in an unvaccinated child with a fine maculo-papular rash and fever includes rubella and measles

Sacral bed sores can erode down the bone. A polymicrobial bacteraemia may arise from such a site

Cellulitis and abscess formation may arise at injection sites of i.v. drug users. *Staphylococcus aureus* and **streptococci** are important here

Venous ulcers are often colonized by bacteria

The hairline along with throat, nares, axillae, groin, perineum, and wrists can be important sites for **MRSA** carriage

In post-operative wound infections *Staphylococcus aureus* (and **MRSA**) are important

Cat and dog bites can cause severe infection. Penicillin sensitive *Pasteurella multocida* is an organism to consider

Crepitus around the site of a recent colostomy may indicate synergistic necrotizing fasciitis due to polymicrobial infection

Severe cellulitis may arise after months or years in patients who have had saphenous veins removed for CABG

In diabetics, foot ulcers can erode down to the bone. The resulting osteomyelitis may be polymicrobial

247 Some of the important clinical situations involved in infection of the skin and soft tissue. (CABG: coronary artery by-pass graft.)

at 30°C, the optimum growth temperature for this organism. Some examples of bone and joint infections are shown in **248**. Advances in orthopaedic surgery make joint replacement a common practice. Infections of prosthetic joints may necessitate removal of the device.

In addition to local infections, the skin is an important site for the manifestation of systemic disease, and it should be carefully examined. Some of the terms used to classify skin lesions are shown in **249**. Small, non-blanching lesions progressing to larger petechial and then ecchymotic lesions must prompt the consideration of meningococcal sepsis. In the immunosuppressed patient, new skin lesions should be seen by the dermatologist and, as necessary, biopsied and sent for histological and microbiological investigation. Organisms can be deposited in the skin from a focus elsewhere in the body. Unusual organisms such as the fungus fusarium may be isolated, clearly influencing the management of the patient.

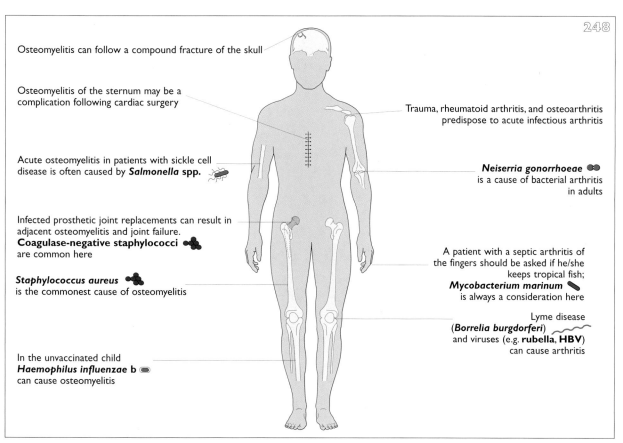

Osteomyelitis can follow a compound fracture of the skull

Osteomyelitis of the sternum may be a complication following cardiac surgery

Acute osteomyelitis in patients with sickle cell disease is often caused by **Salmonella spp.**

Infected prosthetic joint replacements can result in adjacent osteomyelitis and joint failure. **Coagulase-negative staphylococci** are common here

Staphylococcus aureus is the commonest cause of osteomyelitis

In the unvaccinated child **Haemophilus influenzae b** can cause osteomyelitis

Trauma, rheumatoid arthritis, and osteoarthritis predispose to acute infectious arthritis

Neiserria gonorrhoeae is a cause of bacterial arthritis in adults

A patient with a septic arthritis of the fingers should be asked if he/she keeps tropical fish; **Mycobacterium marinum** is always a consideration here

Lyme disease (**Borrelia burgdorferi**) and viruses (e.g. **rubella**, **HBV**) can cause arthritis

248 Examples of infections of the joints and bone.

249 The differentiation of macules, papules, vesicles, and pustules.

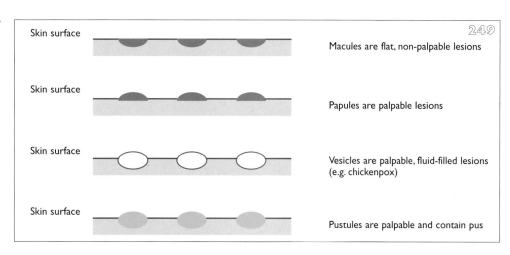

Skin surface — Macules are flat, non-palpable lesions

Skin surface — Papules are palpable lesions

Skin surface — Vesicles are palpable, fluid-filled lesions (e.g. chickenpox)

Skin surface — Pustules are palpable and contain pus

Organisms

A list of bacteria commonly associated with the various conditions discussed in this chapter is shown in **250**.

Spirochetes such as *Treponema pallidum*, the causative agent of syphilis, and *Borrelia burgdorferi*, the causative agent of Lyme disease, produce skin rashes. Lyme disease is transmitted from animals such as deer by ticks (a zoonosis), and the rash migrates out from the site of the tick bite and is termed erythema migrans. Arthritis is another manifestation of Lyme disease.

A number of viruses have the skin as their target organ. HSV and VZV produce characteristic vesicular lesions. In the case of HSV these lesions are usually restricted to the genital or oral regions, but in chickenpox, lesions are widespread over the upper body, arms, and head. These viruses can persist in the dorsal root ganglia and have the potential to cause reactivated disease. With VZV this presents as shingles or herpes zoster, which has a characteristic dermatomal distribution, depending on which nerve root the latent virus is reactivated from. Measles, rubella, parvovirus B19, and HSV6 produce a characteristic skin rash which is useful in diagnosis.

Pathogenesis
Infections of the skin

An intact skin surface, its relative dryness, desquamation of cells, a surface pH between 5.0 and 6.0, and a normal flora of coagulase-negative staphylococci and other gram-positive bacteria such as the 'diphtheroids' are all barriers to infection. In addition, sebum produced by the sebaceous glands is converted to free fatty acids by the normal flora of the skin, and these fatty acids inhibit the growth of pathogens such as group A streptococcus.

Bacteria enter the skin via minor abrasions, surgical incisions or via the hair follicles. It is likely that conditions such as cellulitis may also arise as a result of an occult bacteraemia. Group A streptococci may enter the blood from the pharynx or from lesions around the toes such as 'athlete's foot', and if they settle in skin where the anatomy and physiology are compromised, cellulitis can arise. This is probably the situation in individuals who have had leg veins removed for cardiac surgery, who later develop cellulitis in the calf. The removal of the veins compromises local anatomy, and mild trauma with bruising may provide a site for an organism such as group A streptococcus to initiate an infection.

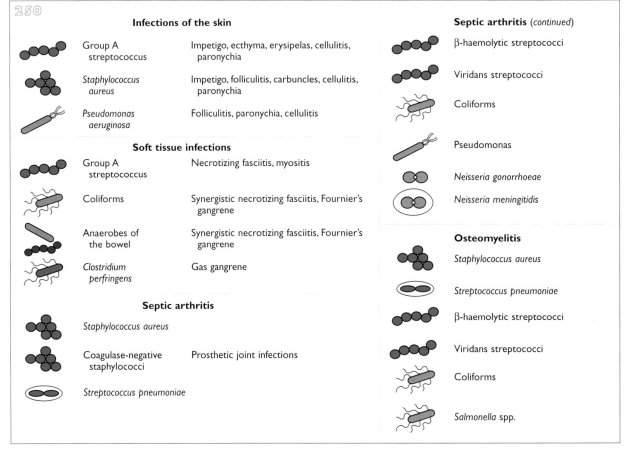

250 Organisms to consider in skin, soft tissue, joint, and bone infections.

An outline of the structure of the skin and a range of skin infections including impetigo, staphylococcal scalded skin syndrome, infection of the hair follicles, ecthyma, erysipelas, and cellulitis is shown in **251a–d**.

Fasciitis and myositis

Necrotizing fasciitis can be caused by an organism such as group A streptococcus alone or by a combination of bacteria acting synergistically. In the latter example, organisms from the bowel flora are usually involved, causing fasciitis of the abdominal wall following surgery.

Bacteria enter the fascial plane beneath the subcutaneous tissue following trauma or surgery. In the case of group A streptococcus, bacteria can reach this site by an occult bacteraemia, and settle in some transient abnormal structure such as a small haematoma following

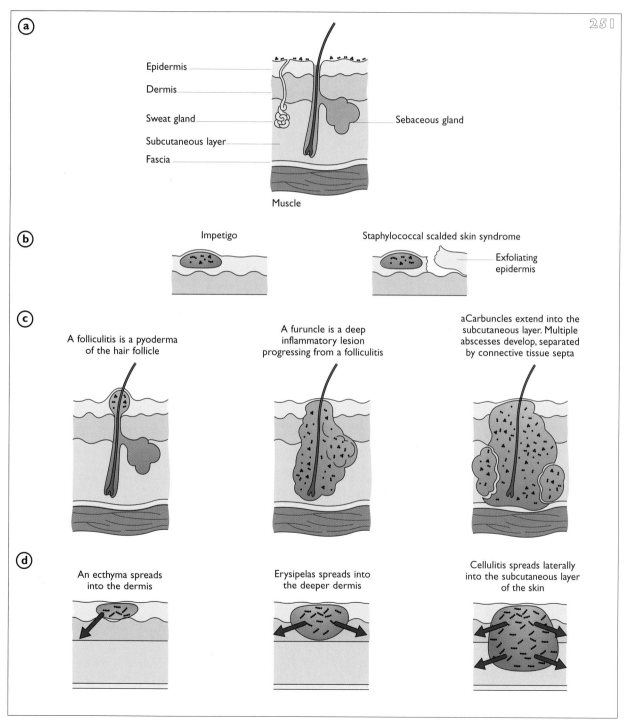

251 (**a**) The structure of the skin. (**b**) Impetigo and staphylococcal scalded skin syndrome. (**c**) Infections in the hair follicles. (**d**) Ecthyma, erysipelas, cellulitis.

bruising. Examination of the limb of a human cadaver shows that there is little resistance to dissection along the fascial planes that separate the skin from muscle. Once bacteria enter the fascial plane, they can spread rapidly, and the resulting inflammatory response then affects the neurovascular bundles lying within the fascial plane.

Thrombosis of the vessels compromises the blood supply and nerves to the skin. The skin over the affected area progresses from a red and painful cellulitic-type picture to a dusky red colour, and it then becomes grey and painless with fluid-filled bullae. Invasion of the deeper fascia and progression to myositis can arise (**252a–d**). It is thus essential that any patient with cellulitis is fully assessed to exclude fasciitis. The later the situation is recognized, the poorer the prognosis. Surgical debridement is essential in preventing the condition deteriorating.

In military conflicts of the past, gas gangrene caused by *Clostridium perfringens* was a common life-threatening condition, arising in devitalized wounds contaminated with soil. Such an environment was ideal for this anaerobe to multiply and, by producing a range of potent histotoxins, gangrene resulted, and amputation was the usual outcome. In more recent military conflicts, modern medicine has reduced gas gangrene to negligible levels. Prompt debridement of devitalized tissue and the practice of leaving wounds open after operation minimize the chance of gangrene arising.

It is probable in synergistic soft tissue infections, where for example an abdominal surgical wound is contaminated with bowel flora, that coliforms use up available oxygen in the tissue, enabling mixed anaerobes to exploit the situation. Factors such as poor nutrition, obesity, and diabetes are likely to contribute to the development of this synergistic gangrene. Fournier's gangrene is a serious soft tissue infection involving the scrotum, which can spread to the abdominal wall. Predisposing factors include local trauma and diabetes. This is a polymicrobial infection, usually involving organisms of the bowel flora.

Septic arthritis

Septic arthritis is more common in a joint affected by rheumatoid disease or where there is a history of trauma; diabetes, old age, and malnutrition can also contribute to the likelihood of infection. An outline of the structure of a joint and routes whereby bacteria can enter a joint is shown in **253**. The synovium lacks a basement membrane and bacteria in an occult bacteraemia can enter the joint space. Their reproduction results in an inflammatory response with invasion of neutrophils into the joint. Damage to the joint can occur; *Staphylococcus aureus* for example produces a chondrocyte protease that can destroy cartilage.

Infections of prosthetic joint devices can arise as a result of organisms such as coagulase-negative staphylococci being introduced at the time of operation or by the haematogenous route (**254**). The inflammatory response gives rise to continual pain, which is exacerbated by movement.

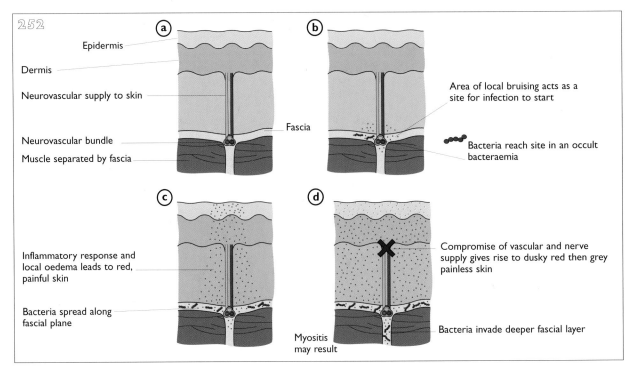

252 The mechanism whereby fasciitis arises. (**a**) Skin and muscle are separated by the fascial plane. (**b**) Bacteria can reach the fascial plane by the blood. (**c**) They spread along the fascial plane. (**d**) The neurovascular supply to the skin and invasion of the deeper fascial planes can occur.

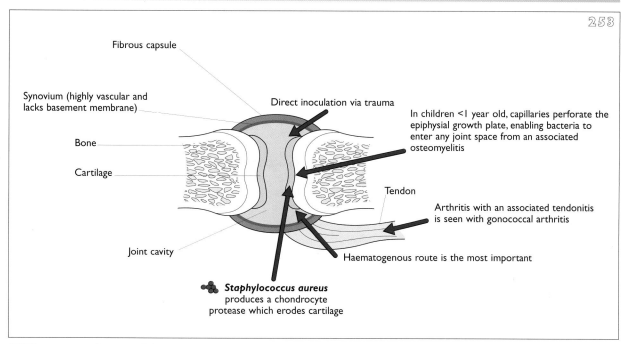

253 The structure of a joint and the routes whereby bacteria reach a joint.

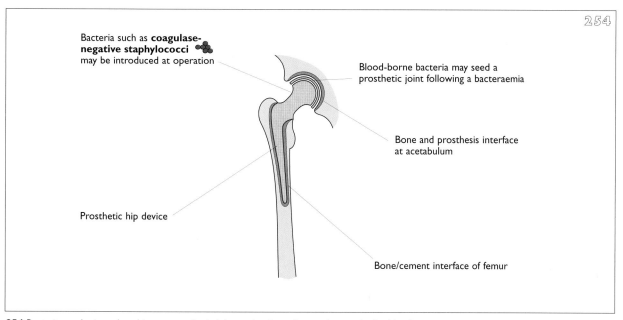

254 Bacteria can be introduced into a prosthetic joint at the time of operation or via the blood.

Osteomyelitis

Bone may become infected following direct introduction of bacteria into this tissue by trauma or surgery. Osteomyelitis can also arise from the haematogenous route. An outline of this process in children is shown in **255**. Capillary loops in the metaphysis of a long bone may develop small haematomas as a result of some external force such as trauma. Organisms from an occult bacteraemia can settle in this haematoma and initiate infection. The resulting medullary abscess can then extend, via the Haversian canal system, through the cortex of the bone. A sequestrum of necrotic tissue remains within the bone.

In children, the fibrous periosteum of the bone is not breached and a sub-periosteal abscess forms. In adults, the periosteum is breached and soft tissue abscesses occur. New bone, termed the involucrum, is laid down around the breach on the surface of the bone. In children less than 1 year of age, the infection in the metaphysis of any bone can erode through the growth plate and cause an associated septic arthritis. After this age an associated septic arthritis only occurs where the joint space encloses the metaphysis, such as the hip joint.

Infection of bone is classed as either acute or chronic. Chronic infection may have continued for weeks and months before the diagnosis is confirmed. Whether acute or chronic, osteomyelitis is a major problem as it is very difficult to eradicate bacteria from the sequestrum, and even in treated acute infection, bacteria may survive in a 'dormant' state to cause disease many years later.

Diagnosis

It is important that any pus from soft tissue, aspirate from a septic joint and blood cultures are collected and sent for microbiological investigation. Blood culture can identify the organism involved in acute osteomyelitis. Radiology, including X-ray and MRI, as well as measurement of CRP and ESR are part of the diagnostic armament. Rising creatinine phosphokinase (CPK) levels can indicate progression of cellulitis to fasciitis and myositis.

Treatment

An outline of some of the antibiotics that can be used is shown in **256**. Superficial skin infections, including mild cellulitis can be treated with a 5–7 day course of an oral antibiotic. Flucloxacillin is reasonable here as it has activity against *Staphylococcus aureus* and group A streptococcus. In moderate to severe cellulitis, intravenous antibiotics must be given, at least in the initial stages of treatment. Septic arthritis may require antibiotics for 4 weeks, acute osteomyelitis 6 weeks, and chronic osteomyelitis in excess of 3 months.

Public health issues

Skin carriage of *Staphylococcus aureus*, including MRSA, is well known. The importance of the latter organism is well recognized in the hospital setting, where it can be a significant infection control problem. It is recognized that MRSA also exists in the community, and that it circulates between the hospital and the community as part of the

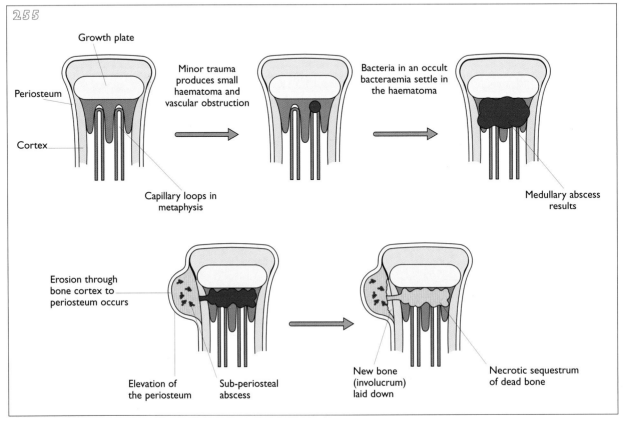

255 The mechanisms whereby osteomyelitis develops in a child.

normal flora of individuals. Group A streptococcus may cause outbreaks of pyoderma in the community, usually in the setting of groups of people who have close contact with each other, such as in schools.

Both these examples can be used to highlight infection control issues. The mainstay of infection control is a clean environment, prompt identification of the infected patient, and good practice by the health care worker. Hand washing is the key to all of this, and it is essential that this basic practice is performed on every necessary occasion.

Comment

When aspirating fluid from a joint, it is essential to use scrupulous aseptic technique. In the setting of the patient who may have an infected prosthetic joint, the orthopaedic surgeon must be contacted to review the patient and collect any specimens. Introduction of bacteria into such a joint by an unskilled health care worker can have disastrous consequences.

In the management of an infected prosthetic joint such as a total knee replacement (TKR), it essential that the orthopaedic surgeon and medical microbiologist work together. At operation and after removal of the prosthesis, at least six biopsies should be taken from within the joint. These should also be inoculated into enrichment culture to ensure that bacteria present are given every opportunity to grow. Once the organism has been identified, and its antibiotic susceptibility pattern determined, the patient should have 4–6 weeks of antibiotics. As gram-positive bacteria such as the coagulase-negative staphylococci are usually isolated, intravenous teicoplanin on a daily basis and oral RIF are a useful combination as they can be used in the community setting, and the patient is thus discharged home.

After this period, the patient has no antibiotics for 2–3 weeks, then at operation, biopsies are again taken before reimplantation of the prosthesis. If the biopsy specimens do not grow the original or any other organism, no further antibiotics are given. If the same organism is grown, antibiotics are given for 3 months. Tetracyclines, RIF, and new agents such as linezolid that can all be given by mouth are useful here. If a patient has a further infected prosthesis, antibiotics may have to be given indefinitely, particularly in the older patient.

There is no consensus as to when to give antibiotic prophylaxis to patients who have a prosthetic joint and are undergoing, for example, dental treatment. At the very least, antibiotics similar to those used to prevent endocarditis should be given if dental treatment occurs within the 3 month period after joint replacement. Local advice and recent recommendations should be sought here.

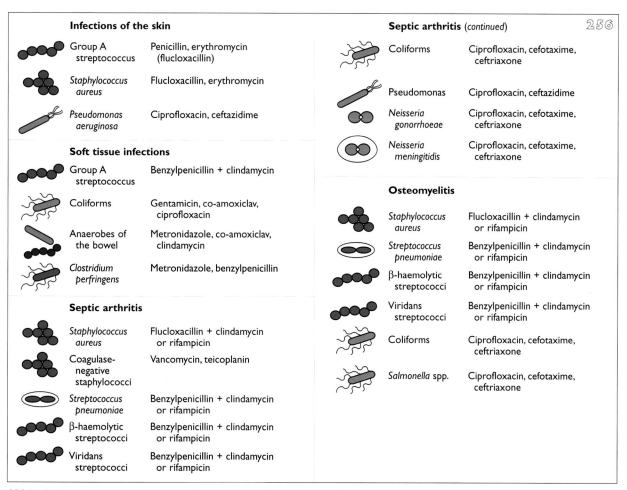

256 Antibiotics that can be used to treat infections of the soft tissue, joint, and bone.

14 Infections in a Modern Society

Introduction

This chapter is concerned with infections in the IVDU, the patient on the ICU and, amongst others, those individuals who are immunosuppressed as a result of chemotherapy given to combat a malignancy. Certain viruses are mentioned here, as an appreciation of them is relevant in the overall assessment of the patients considered in this chapter. For example, the very nature of sharing needles means that the blood-borne viruses HBV, hepatitis C virus, and HIV must always be considered in the IVDU.

Major advances in renal medicine, solid organ transplantation surgery, haematology, and oncology have centred on practices that result in suppression of the immune system. These include the use of steroids and agents such as cyclosporin and tacrolimus. Cyclosporin acts by reducing IL-2 levels and inhibits T cell proliferation and activation of cytotoxic T cells. This suppression of cell-mediate immunity (CMI) brings to the fore organisms which would normally be controlled by a competent CMI system.

The members of the Herpesviridae, including HSV, CMV, EBV, and VZV are an important group of organisms. Being DNA-containing viruses, they have the potential for persistence after primary infection, and reactivated infection is a problem in the immunosuppressed patient. Bacteria that grow intracellularly within macrophages are also important and include TB, legionella, and listeria. Soil and environmental organisms such as the branching gram-positive bacterium *Nocardia asteroides*, the fungi *Aspergillus fumigatus* and *Pneumocystis carinii*, and parasites such as *Toxoplasma gondii* also need to be considered. The effect of long-term immunosuppression compromises humoral (antibody-mediated) immunity, and bacteria such as *Streptococcus pneumoniae* are always a threat. Common organisms considered in this chapter are shown in **257**.

	IVDU	HD	CAPD	SOT	L/O		IVDU	HD	CAPD	SOT	L/O
Staphylococcus aureus	✓	✓	✓	✓	✓	*Cryptococcus neoformans*				✓	✓
Coagulase-negative staphylococci		✓	✓	✓	✓	*Pneumocystis carinii*				✓	✓
Streptococci	✓	✓	✓	✓	✓	*Toxoplasma gondii*				✓	✓
Enterococci		✓	✓	✓	✓	HSV, CMV, EBV, VZV				✓S	✓S
Coliforms		✓	✓	✓	✓	HIV	✓	✓S		✓S	✓
Pseudomonas aeruginosa		✓	✓	✓	✓	HCV	✓	✓S		✓S	✓
Anaerobes	✓			✓	✓	HBV	✓	✓S		✓S	✓
Legionella pneumophila				✓	✓						
Listeria monocytogenes				✓	✓						
Nocardia asteroides				✓	✓						
Aspergillus fumigatus				✓	✓						
Candida spp.	✓	✓	✓	✓	✓						

257 A list of the organisms that should be considered in the individuals discussed in this chapter. (IVDU: intravenous drug user; HD: haemodialysis patient; CAPD: chronic ambulatory peritoneal dialysis patient; SOT: solid organ transplant patient; L/O: leukaemic/oncology patient. S: patients would usually be screened for these viruses; HSV; herpes simplex virus; CMV: cytomegalovirus; EBV: Epstein Barr virus; VZV: varicella zoster virus; HIV: human immunodeficiency virus; HCV: hepatitis C virus; HBV: hepatitis B virus.)

Although HIV is not covered in this book, it is important to recognize that many of the infections discussed here in relation to the immunosuppressed haematology, oncology, or organ-transplant patient are also relevant in HIV infected individuals. This underlies some of the similarities in the effect of HIV infection and iatrogenic immunosuppression.

In addition to traditional laboratory methods in diagnosis, new molecular methods have now become essential in the diagnosis of infection in the immunocompromised patient. Nucleic acid tests such the PCR are the cornerstone of these new techniques and are of particular use in the diagnosis of viral infections. In addition, quantitative PCR for CMV, HIV, and HBV is available and can be used to monitor the effect of specific antiviral chemotherapy.

This chapter ends with a short section on biological warfare and bio-terrorism, a most unfortunate fact in this modern world.

Intravenous drug user

For the IVDU, social exclusion, poverty, malnutrition, and drug use all contribute to weakening the individual's immune status. Repeated injections into the groin to access the femoral vein compromise the integrity of the skin and soft tissues. Repeated introduction of bacteria from the flora of the groin gives rise to cellulitis and abscess formation; septic thrombophlebitis of the femoral vein can also occur. *Staphylococcus aureus*, streptococci of the *Streptococcus anginosus* group, and anaerobes should always be considered in these infections.

It is likely that injected drugs contain particulate impurities which, travelling at speed, impinge on and damage the endothelium of the tricuspid valve. The resulting deposition of fibrin and platelets at this site is ideal for bacteria in the blood to settle in and initiate endocarditis. Microbial contamination of drugs can also be a major issue. *Clostridium novyi* is one example and it can cause fulminating systemic infection.

Some of the common sites of infection and organisms to consider in the IVDU are shown in **258**. Blood cultures should be collected, and any tissue or pus that is obtained should be examined promptly in the laboratory. Acute endocarditis is a medical emergency, and after the collection of several sets of blood cultures over a 20–30 minute period, high dose antibiotics appropriate for *Staphylococcus aureus* must be given. Urgent referral to the cardiothoracic surgeons should be made in the setting of deteriorating cardiac function.

The prescription of antibiotics in this group of patients can be a problem. Peripheral intravenous access is usually difficult as veins are often fibrosed as a result of repeated drug injection and a central line may be needed. This may create a further problem, as the IVDU now has a direct route to inject illicit drugs brought in to hospital by friends or relatives. This can be of particular concern when the patient has just had a valve replaced for infective endocarditis. The physician and medical microbiologist need to consult regularly on the best regime for each individual patient and consider the use of antibiotics which have good oral bioavailability.

The patient who is HBV, HCV, or HIV positive needs to be referred to the GUM physicians for appropriate management. Follow-up of contacts who may be at risk of acquiring these viruses is needed.

Intensive care patient

There are many reasons for patients being admitted to an ICU. Severe community acquired pneumonia and meningococcal sepsis are examples. Patients admitted to the cardiothoracic ICU after routine heart surgery usually require less than 24 hours of intensive care to stabilize them, which is essentially ventilatory support.

Septic shock was referred to in chapter 5, and is relevant to this section as well. As an example, the patient who has had surgery following a ruptured abdominal abscess may have a prolonged stay on ICU. In addition to ventilatory support, cardiac and renal support is an essential part of their management. These patients are often described as being 'septic', and while the organisms of the bowel may be relevant in the first few days of treatment, the presence of a continuing systemic inflammatory response syndrome (SIRS) becomes the main problem. The longer the support for the multi-organ failure arising from this inflammatory insult is needed, the less likely the outcome will be favourable. In addition, it is reasonable to assume that such patients become immunosuppressed as the derangement of their immune system continues.

The other problem that faces the patient is the intensity of the care itself. The ETT used for ventilation provides a direct route for bacteria to enter the lungs. The ongoing requirement for arterial and venous access provides a route for bacteria to initiate line infections and line-associated bacteraemia. A naso-gastric tube can obstruct the opening of a nasal sinus, with sinusitis resulting. Permanent catheterization of the bladder provides a route for bacteria and yeasts to enter the body. Bacteria isolated from blood, venous and arterial access sites, endotracheal tubes, or urine should be used to guide treatment. The medical microbiologist should provide this information by a ward-based service and take part in the decisions about the antibiotics to use in each patient.

While the antibiotics given to the patient on admission to the unit may be appropriate, other organisms continually need to be considered. These include yeasts, pseudomonas, MRSA, and multi-resistant gram-negative bacteria such as *Klebsiella pneumoniae*. In the ICU setting, isolates of the latter organism resistant to all the cephalosporins, gentamicin, and ciprofloxacin can be found. Clearly the treatment options available for such an organism are reduced and centre on the carbapenems. The reason why such bacteria are resistant to all the cephalosporins is that they produce plasmid-mediated extended spectrum β-lactamases (ESBLs) that can inactivate all these agents.

Antibiotics used on ICU include piperacillin/tazobactam and the carbapenems, usually combined with an aminoglycoside. When a new course of antibiotics is instituted, it should be reviewed after 4 days, and if the patient has improved the antibiotics may be discontinued. If there is no improvement the regime should be continued

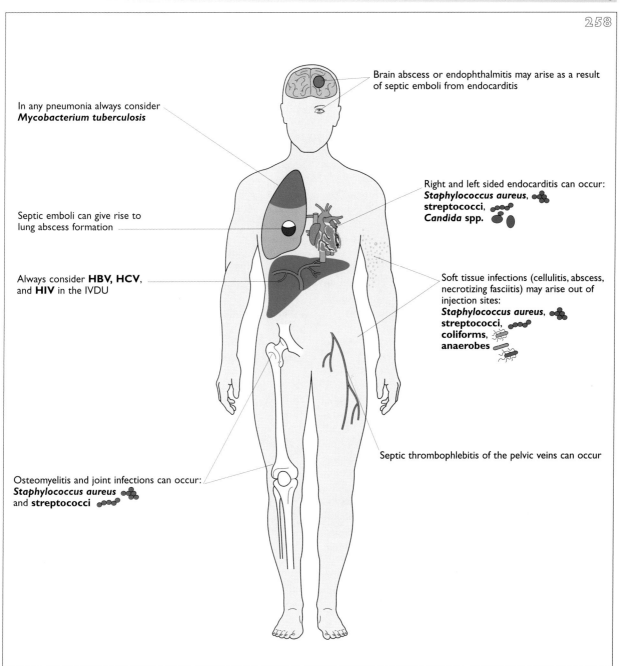

Brain abscess or endophthalmitis may arise as a result of septic emboli from endocarditis

In any pneumonia always consider *Mycobacterium tuberculosis*

Septic emboli can give rise to lung abscess formation

Always consider **HBV, HCV**, and **HIV** in the IVDU

Right and left sided endocarditis can occur: *Staphylococcus aureus*, **streptococci**, *Candida* spp.

Soft tissue infections (cellulitis, abscess, necrotizing fasciitis) may arise out of injection sites: *Staphylococcus aureus*, **streptococci**, **coliforms**, **anaerobes**

Septic thrombophlebitis of the pelvic veins can occur

Osteomyelitis and joint infections can occur: *Staphylococcus aureus* and **streptococci**

258 Some of the sites and organisms to consider in the intravenous drug user.

or changed to other agents. In the setting of the deteriorating patient with abdominal sepsis for example, and when yeasts are isolated from a sterile site, or from two sites such as urine and respiratory secretions, antifungal agents such as fluconazole or a lipid-based form of amphotericin B must be considered.

Immunocompromised patient
Splenectomized patient
Splenectomized individuals are at risk of overwhelming infection by encapsulated bacteria such as *Streptococcus pneumoniae*, *Neisseria meningitidis*, and *Haemophilus influenzae* b. The spleen is an important site of functioning macrophages, and it is an integral part of the humoral (antibody producing) immune system needed for the control of these encapsulated bacteria. All splenectomized individuals should be vaccinated against these bacteria. Following loss of the spleen they should also be placed on a prophylactic antibiotic, which is usually oral penicillin. Children should take the antibiotic until they reach the age of 16 years at least, and adults should continue to take the antibiotic for at least 2 years after splenectomy.

Perhaps the most important action is for these individuals to carry a medical alert card or bracelet stating their condition. Any health care worker can then be alerted if the person presents with symptoms and signs of infection compatible with the organisms cited above. A major function of the spleen is to remove damaged or abnormal RBC from circulation. When splenectomized individuals travel to areas of the world where malaria is endemic they must be warned of their increased risk. In addition to antimalarial prophylaxis, contact with mosquitoes must be minimized by use of nets and repellent sprays.

Renal dialysis patient
Haemodialysis
Patients on haemodialysis are at risk of infection at the site where a dialysis catheter is inserted, such as a great vein of the neck. These long-term lines can become colonized with staphylococci, enterococci, coliforms, pseudomonas, and yeasts, resulting in infection around the insertion site, bacteraemia or fungaemia. Any fluid around the site, as well as peripheral and central line blood culture sets should be collected.

In haemodialysis patients the most important organisms to consider are the blood-borne viruses HBV, HCV, and HIV. All patients on haemodialysis need to be regularly screened for these viruses even though modern dialysis machines are such that cross contamination is unlikely. However, patients who are known to be infected with one or more of these viruses are dialysed on a separate machine. It is now routine practice to give patients on haemodialysis the HBV vaccine. The overall response to the vaccine may not be particularly good, reflecting the immunosuppressed nature of these patients in chronic renal failure.

Chronic ambulatory peritoneal dialysis peritonitis
CAPD has been one of the major advances in the management of patients with end-stage renal failure, allowing patients to be managed at home. CAPD peritonitis is a recognized complication of the process, and up to half of patients on CAPD will have an episode of peritonitis in the first year. Recurrent infection may result in termination of CAPD in certain patients, necessitating their return to haemodialysis.

CAPD peritonitis arises as a result of several factors. These patients are considered to be immunocompromised as a consequence of their renal failure. However, the most important factor is the disruption of the integrity of the abdominal wall by the long-term catheter passing into the peritoneal cavity. Organisms can enter the peritoneum by subcutaneous passage or they may contaminate the dialysis fluid itself. Dialysis fluid has a low pH and high osmolality, which probably impairs the functioning of macrophages and neutrophils. In addition, the fluid is likely to affect the normal physiology of the bowel, and bacteria may cross the bowel wall into the peritoneum. The repeated changes of the dialysis fluid wash out opsonins such as complement factor C3.

Patients with CAPD peritonitis may present with abdominal pain and tenderness, nausea, and vomiting, and the dialysis fluid is cloudy. At this stage it is usual to prescribe empirical antibiotics by the intraperitoneal route. Either vancomycin or teicoplanin and an aminoglycoside such as gentamicin are given. These antibiotics cover the common bacteria found in CAPD peritonitis. Diagnosis relies on the collection of fluid for microscopy and culture (**259**); the WCC is raised above the normal value of 100/µL and the differential count usually shows a predominance of neutrophils. The gram stain may identify bacteria or yeasts. On occasion there may repeatedly be no growth from the CAPD fluid, and other organisms such as mycobacteria need to be considered. Occasionally algae have been known to contaminate CAPD fluid.

Solid organ transplant patient
Successful transplantation of a solid organ depends on the degree of cross-matching between the donor organ and the recipient, and the extent of the immunosuppression that has to be given in order for the transplanted organ to survive and function. Immunosuppression will put the patient at risk of a wide range of organisms, which include bacteria, fungi, viruses, and parasites. For this reason it is usual for the donor and recipient to be screened serologically for a number of organisms prior to transplantation. Some infections such as HIV in a potential donor are an absolute contraindication to transplantation. In other instances, for example with CMV, a positive donor to negative recipient transplant can be done. Close monitoring for CMV DNA by PCR in the appropriate clinical situation after transplantation would be mandatory so that antiviral treatment with an agent such as ganciclovir can be instituted promptly.

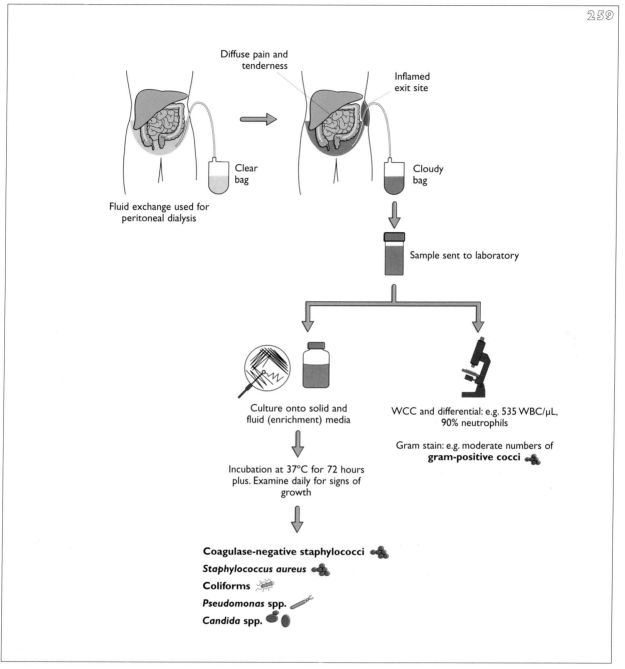

259

Diffuse pain and
tenderness

Inflamed
exit site

Clear
bag

Cloudy
bag

Fluid exchange used for
peritoneal dialysis

Sample sent to laboratory

Culture onto solid and
fluid (enrichment) media

WCC and differential: e.g. 535 WBC/µL,
90% neutrophils

Gram stain: e.g. moderate numbers of
gram-positive cocci

Incubation at 37°C for 72 hours
plus. Examine daily for signs of
growth

Coagulase-negative staphylococci
Staphylococcus aureus
Coliforms
Pseudomonas spp.
Candida spp.

259 Peritonitis in the chronic ambulatory peritoneal dialysis (CAPD) patient. In the setting of symptoms and cloudy bags, CAPD fluid should be sent for microscopy and culture. Some common organisms are shown.

Three points need to be borne in mind in the transplant patient with a fever. These are rejection of the organ, infection, and drug fever. In addition to fever, rejection may be accompanied by myalgia and arthritis and can clearly mimic infection. It is thus important that all possible sites of infection are considered and the appropriate specimens taken. In solid organ transplant patients, infections can in general be divided into those that occur in the first month after the operation and those that occur in the next 5 months or so, the immunosuppressed period (260). In the first month, infections that arise are a result of the transplantation itself and the intensive care period that follows. Surgical wound infections, abscess formation, ventilation-associated pneumonia, bacteraemia arising from long-term central lines, and UTI are examples. For each type of transplant, local complications may arise. In renal transplantation, infection in the urinary tract is a recognized complication. In liver transplantation, liver and peritoneal abscesses can occur. These relate to the

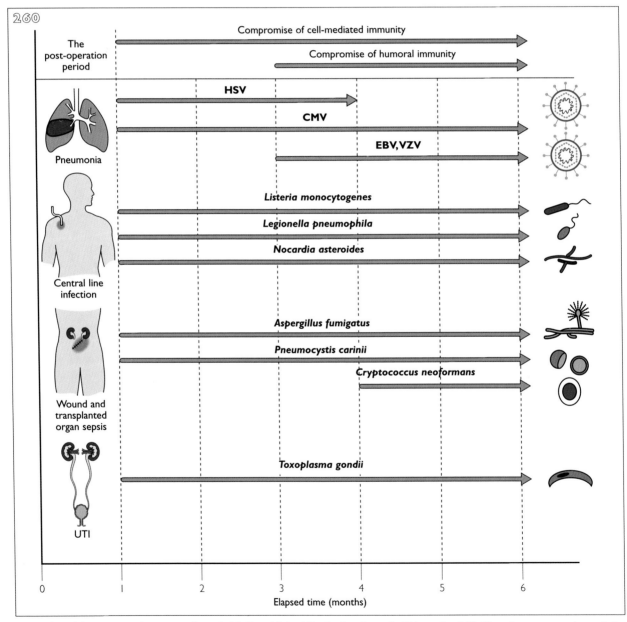

260 In the solid organ transplant patient the main infection risk is within the first 6 months. This can be divided into the post-operative period and the immunocompromised period. Relevant clinical situations and organisms are shown. (CMV: cytomegalovirus; EBV: Epstein Barr virus; HSV: herpes simplex virus; UTI: urinary tract infection; VZV: varicella zoster virus.) (Modified, with permission from Rubin RH *et al.* (1981) Infection in the renal transplant recipient. *American Journal of Medicine* **70**, 406.)

various anastomoses that have to be made including re-routing of the biliary tract drainage. In heart and lung transplantation, mediastinitis can be a problem. The anastomoses of the lung and the ablation of the cough reflex are all important contributors to infection here.

Haematology and oncology patient

In this group of patients the neutropenic leukaemic patient exemplifies the challenges in the diagnosis and treatment of infection. Within 4 or 5 days of initiation of induction chemotherapy, the neutrophil count in these patients drops below 1000/μL. In the ensuing neutropenic period the patient is at risk of overwhelming infection. Clearly the chemotherapy is not only acting on bone marrow, but all high turnover cells of the body will be affected, and mucositis of the upper gastrointestinal tract is an example. Some possible sites of infection in the neutropenic patient are identified in **261**.

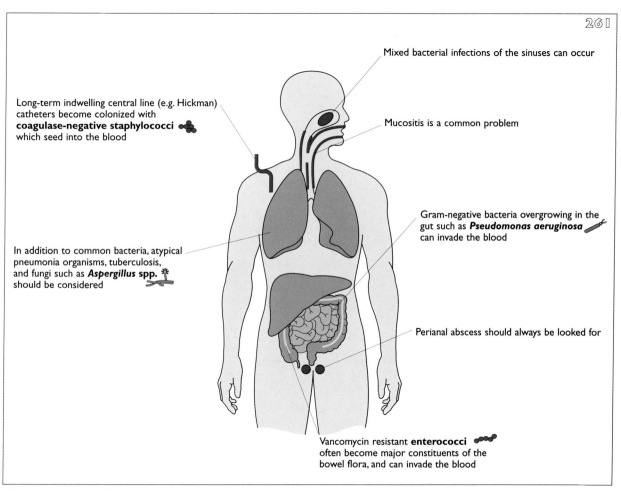

261

Mixed bacterial infections of the sinuses can occur

Long-term indwelling central line (e.g. Hickman) catheters become colonized with **coagulase-negative staphylococci** which seed into the blood

Mucositis is a common problem

Gram-negative bacteria overgrowing in the gut such as *Pseudomonas aeruginosa* can invade the blood

In addition to common bacteria, atypical pneumonia organisms, tuberculosis, and fungi such as *Aspergillus* spp. should be considered

Perianal abscess should always be looked for

Vancomycin resistant **enterococci** often become major constituents of the bowel flora, and can invade the blood

261 Some sites where infection can arise in the neutropenic leukaemic patient.

Haematology units will have specific protocols for the empirical treatment of fever in the neutropenic patient (**262a–c**). These can be influenced by microbiology results, of which blood culture is the most important. Usually a combination of a broad-spectrum agent such as piperacillin/tazobactam combined with an aminoglycoside is used first. If the temperature does not settle within 48–72 hours, this should be replaced with vancomycin and ceftazidime. A glycopeptide is given here to ensure cover for possible colonization of long-term indwelling lines by staphylococci. After this there should be a fairly low index of suspicion of fungal infection, and candida and aspergillus are relevant. Aspergillus infection in the lungs and other organs has a poorer outcome and imaging of the lung must be done to identify cavitating lesions. Amphotericin B, usually in some lipid carriage form, is

given. The significant use of glycopeptide antibiotics itself produces another problem, and that is the selection of bacteria such as VRE.

Biological warfare and bio-terrorism

The deliberate use of infectious agents in warfare and terrorism is now part of modern society. The indiscriminate use of such agents can have a devastating potential to disrupt both military and civilian life. In order to be effective, an agent has to have certain properties. It has to be stable so that it can survive in the environment for long periods without being inactivated; the spore-forming gram-positive *Bacillus anthracis* is one example. The infecting dose of the agent has to be small. One microgram of the toxin of *Clostridium botulinum* can be lethal, and the infecting dose of shigella is in the order of 100 organisms. The agent should be

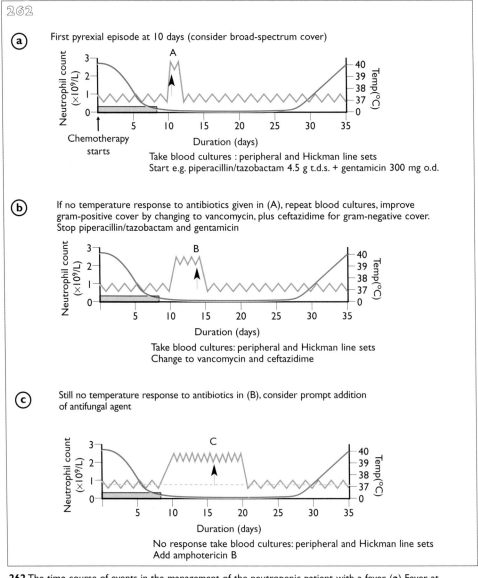

262 The time course of events in the management of the neutropenic patient with a fever. (**a**) Fever at day 10 [A] is treated with a broad-spectrum agent and gentamicin. (**b**) When there is no response, antibiotics are changed [B], with vancomycin being given for possible staphylococcal line infection. (**c**) If there is still no response an antifungal agent should be added [C].

contagious, spreading easily through the population. The pneumonic form of the plague organism *Yersinia pestis* is one agent that is highly contagious. There should not be an effective vaccine to prevent illness and the organism has to be easy to produce and introduce into a susceptible human population. It is fortunate that currently no one agent satisfies all these criteria. Even so there is potential for considerable concern about the use of such weapons, and an index of suspicion with any unusual clinical presentation has to be entertained, especially when two or more individuals are affected.

Bacillus anthracis

Anthrax is a disease that occurs in herbivores such as the wild ungulates, sheep, and cattle. Human cases in countries where the disease is more common are usually found in agricultural workers or those involved in processing animal leather and hair. In the setting of bio-terrorism, parcels and letters contaminated with the spores of the bacterium have caused disease. The bacterium grows well on simple laboratory media. Under unfavourable conditions, *Bacillus anthracis* produces a heat-stable spore. The vegetative cell produces a polypeptide capsule and exotoxin, both of which are required for full virulence. The exotoxin has three components, protective antigen (PA) which binds the toxin to the surface of eucaryotic cells, oedema factor (EF) which acts as an adenylcyclase inside cells, and lethal factor (LF) which has an enzymatic role in the cell. None of the components of the exotoxin are active on their own, but together cause rapid cell death.

There are three forms of clinical anthrax: 1) cutaneous is where the spores are introduced into an abrasion in the skin and the reproducing vegetative bacteria incite a local inflammatory response; 2); inhalation anthrax probably requires an infecting dose in the order of 10^4 spores. However, once this form of disease develops, its rapid progression means that the outcome is poor; 3) gastrointestinal disease can also occur, with invasion and ulceration of the gastrointestinal tract.

Isolates of *Bacillus anthracis* are usually sensitive to penicillin and ciprofloxacin. A vaccine which contains inactivated exotoxin is available.

Botulism

The toxin of *Clostridium botulinum* is one of the most potent toxins known, with 1 µg being lethal. There are a number of antigenically different toxins, designated A through to G, with E being the most potent. The toxin is inactivated by boiling, but may be stable in tap water for several days, especially if exposure to air and alkaline conditions is minimized. Botulism is food or water-borne. Nausea, vomiting, abdominal pain, and cranial nerve palsies such as dysphagia and dysphonia, occur within 12–36 hours of ingestion. Rapid respiratory paralysis and death may be the outcome in untreated cases.

Smallpox (variola)

Smallpox is a pox virus, and a member of one of the few DNA-containing virus families which replicate in the cytoplasm of the infected cell. The term smallpox was used in ancient times to distinguish it from giantpox or syphilis.

Smallpox is a disease of humans only, and by the use of an effective vaccine it was eliminated from the world by 1977. Following this, vaccination was stopped in 1978, and legal stocks of the virus were held only in Atlanta in the United States of America and in Moscow. Illegal stores of this virus must be present in other countries.

Although considered to be a contagious organism, it is probably slowly spreading, but overall mortality rates in previous outbreaks have been 30% or higher. The problem now is that the human population is susceptible, as very few individuals are vaccinated. However, prompt and careful identification of cases and vaccination of contacts can limit spread of this virus.

The virus is spread by the respiratory route. A primary viraemia occurs following multiplication of the virus in the lungs. Seeding of the virus and its replication in the liver, spleen, and lymph nodes results in a secondary viraemia, from where the final target organ, the skin, is reached. After an incubation period of 8–18 days, smallpox manifests with marked fever, headache, chills, and malaise, followed by the progressive skin rash.

Discussion

The essential message from this chapter is that the patients involved may be infected with any of a vast range of bacteria, viruses, fungi, and parasites, many of which would not usually be considered as pathogens in the immunocompetent individual. Unusual parasites need to be considered. In the past, patients in the United States have been infected with the trypanosome, *Trypanosoma cruzi*, following heart transplantation. This parasite is endemic in certain parts of Central and South America. In these cases it was not recognized that the heart came from a donor who was chronically infected with this parasite. Other parasites such as *Strongyloides stercoralis* may need to be considered. Wound botulism is now recognised in the IVDU. Any person with a history of drug use who presents with a descending paralysis should alert the diagnosis.

Any unusual skin lesion in an immunosuppressed patient should be assessed for biopsy and the specimen sent for histological and microbiological investigation. It is important that the physician dealing with the patient liaises closely with the infectious diseases physician and medical microbiologist, so that the correct diagnostic procedures and treatments are considered at all times.

Comment

In the United Kingdom, a useful reference document regarding screening in transplantation is cited below. All haematology and medical microbiology departments should have this:

Advisory Committee on the Microbiological Safety of Blood and Tissues for Transplantation (2000). Guidance on the microbiological safety of human organs, tissues and cells in transplantation.

15 Control of Infection in the Hospital and the Community

Introduction

Control of an infection in an individual relies on clinical assessment, the appropriate use of radiological and laboratory resources to aid the diagnosis, and the correct use of antibiotics. The antibiotics should be appropriate for the organisms under consideration, and need to be given at the correct dose and by the appropriate route of administration. The length of the antibiotic regime depends on the clinical situation and can be 3 days in the case of an uncomplicated UTI, 4 weeks for infective endocarditis and 6 months for pulmonary TB.

The responsible and educated use of antibiotics in hospitals and the community must be part of standard clinical practice. Antibiotic prescription is an art, based on a sound knowledge of microbiology. Inappropriate antibiotic use gives rise to many problems, including adverse drug reactions, antibiotic-associated diarrhoea, and antibiotic resistant bacteria. It is also a waste of money.

Continuing use of an antibiotic can lead to the selection of bacteria that are resistant to that agent. When examined over time, this effect can be dramatic. The percentage of *Staphylococcus aureus* isolates from blood culture and CSF in England and Wales that are resistant to methicillin (MRSA), has changed dramatically in the 1990s (**263**). In 1990 it would have been reasonable to give flucloxacillin to a patient with a suspected *Staphylococcus aureus* bacteraemia. By 2001, when MRSA accounted for over 40% of *Staphylococcus aureus* isolates from blood and CSF, the position is not so clear. In a surgical ward where the incidence of MRSA is high, it would be prudent to start treatment with a glycopeptide in a patient with a suspected staphylococcal bacteraemia. This regime can be modified the next day, when the identity and susceptibility profile of the organism is known. The effect of increased use of vancomycin and teicoplanin leads in turn to the selection of vancomycin resistant enterococci (VRE) and *Staphylococcus aureus* with reduced susceptibility to glycopeptides (GISA).

The increasing prevalence of resistant bacteria is an international problem. For example, in the USA MRSA accounted for 30.1% of all *Staphylococcus aureus* isolates in the hospital setting in 1996; by 2000 this had increased to 45.7% (Jones ME *et al.* [2002]. Prevalence of oxacillin resistance in *Staphylococcus aureus* among inpatients and outpatients in the United States in 2000. *Antimicrobial Agents and Chemotherapy* **46**: 3104–05). This study also showed that in the community the prevalence of MRSA changed from 17.3% in 1996 to 28.6% in 2000, emphasizing that resistant bacteria are an issue in both community and hospital. Good antibiotic prescribing and infection control practices thus have to be co-ordinated across the various health care settings in order for any control strategies to have a meaningful outcome.

Antibiotic guidelines

Every hospital and community health care practice should have antibiotic guidelines that can be used for the majority of clinical situations where infection is likely. These guidelines should inform the doctor about the specimens that need to be collected and the antibiotic that should be given. The selection of particular antibiotics must take into account allergies to β-lactam antibiotics, as well as the patient's renal and liver function. When bacteria are subsequently isolated from specimens, their identity and

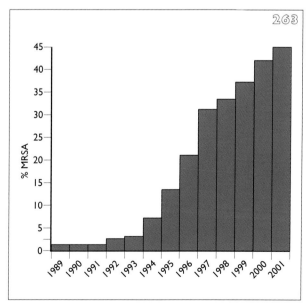

263 The percentage of *Staphylococcus aureus* isolated from blood and CSF in England and Wales that were resistant to methicillin (MRSA) 1989–2001.

susceptibility profile must be used to determine further management. For example, the identification of MRSA in blood culture would warrant a change from flucloxacillin to either vancomycin or teicoplanin. This patient on a surgical ward should preferably be nursed in a side room. At the very least the identification of MRSA should alert all health care workers dealing with the patient to use scrupulous infection control practices.

An outline of a set of simple antibiotic guidelines for a hospital is shown in **264**. It is important to ensure that the correct specimens are collected and sent to the laboratory, preferably before antibiotics have been given. Where there is any doubt about the antibiotics to use, the medical microbiologist or infectious diseases physician must be consulted. Both these specialities practise consultant-led, ward-based microbiology, and if a comprehensive service is not available in a hospital, explanations should be sought from the hospital management.

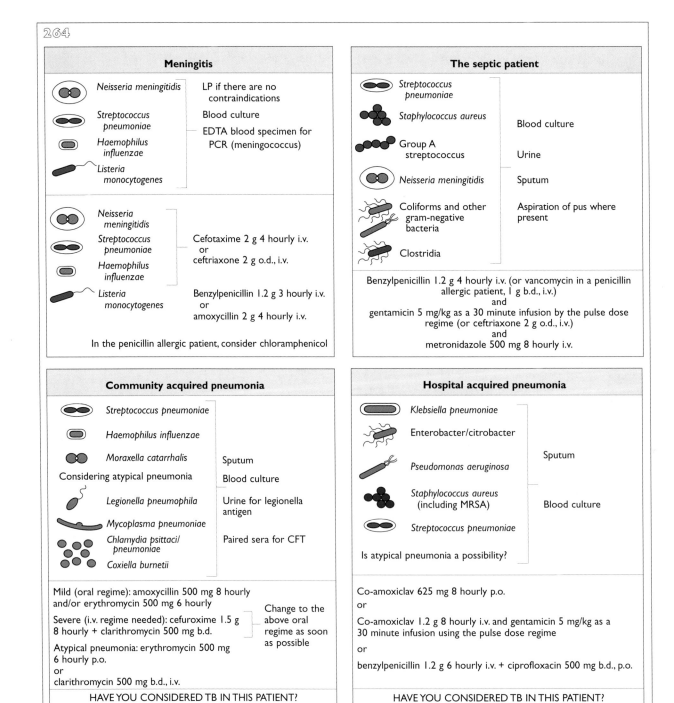

264 Examples of hospital antibiotic guidelines that can be used for adult patients with community or hospital acquired infections.

Prophylactic antibiotics

Prophylactic antibiotics can be given for several reasons. One would be the long-term use of penicillin in the individual who had a splenectomy. The antibiotic reduces the possibility of overwhelming infection with pneumococcus or meningococcus. Individuals with heart valve or other cardiac lesions who are at risk of developing endocarditis should be assessed for antibiotic prophylaxis before any dental or invasive procedure. The most frequent use of prophylactic antibiotics is to prevent infection arising as a result of surgery. The skin is an excellent barrier to infection, and once this is breached, bacteria, often derived from the normal flora of the patient, can be introduced into the surgical wound.

Post-operative wound infection is a major issue in hospitals. They cause morbidity (and mortality), and add significantly to the length and thus cost of a stay in hospital. In order to reduce the chance of a post-operative wound

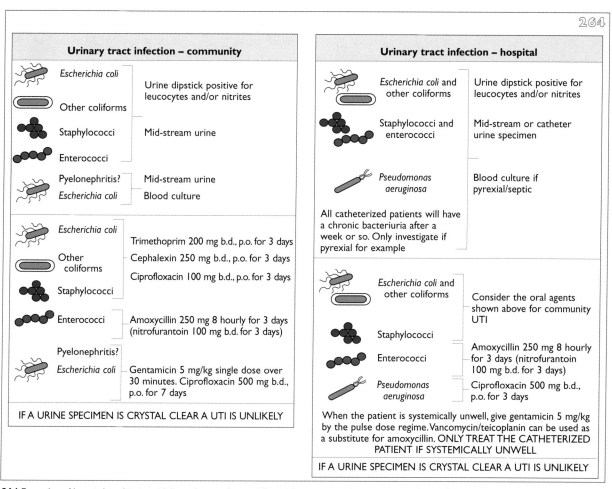

264 Examples of hospital antibiotic guidelines that can be used for adult patients with community or hospital acquired infections (*continued*).

infection, an antibiotic is often used during the procedure. An important aspect of prophylaxis is that if high levels of the antibiotic are present, the chance of any introduced bacteria surviving is minimized. The relative effectiveness of a single dose of an antibiotic such as the cephalosporin cephazolin in preventing infection in relation to the time of operation is shown in **265**. This shows two important points. First, that the levels should be high during the procedure, and second that repeated doses of antibiotic after operation are of decreasing value. If an operation is prolonged, a further dose can be given; antibiotic prophylaxis should not exceed 12–24 hours. The practice of continuing prophylaxis for days is essentially bad practice, and only adds to the selection of resistant bacteria.

A hospital may use the cephalosporin cephazolin for prophylaxis, as this antibiotic is appropriate for MSSA and streptococci, which are the main organisms to consider in wound infection. A number of factors influence the chance of wound infection arising, and this is shown in **266a, b**. A 45-year-old man has a coronary bypass operation and spends 1 day in the ICU. The central line is removed promptly. He carries MSSA in his groin and axillae; cephazolin prevents the few bacteria introduced at operation from causing a problem. An obese 60-year-old man with COAD has the same operation. He requires 10 days of ventilatory support in the ICU, his sternotomy wound needs to be re-opened to drain a haematoma and he carries MRSA in his axilla. The difficult post-operative period and the fact that he carries MRSA, for which cephazolin will not be of use, all add to the likelihood of wound infection involving MRSA.

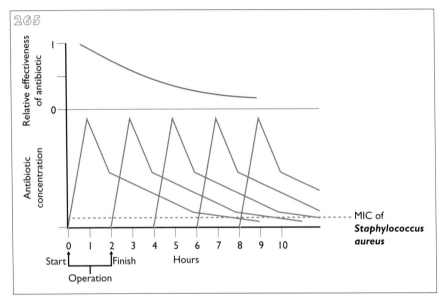

265 The effectiveness of a single dose of a prophylactic antibiotic is progressively diminished if it is given after a procedure.

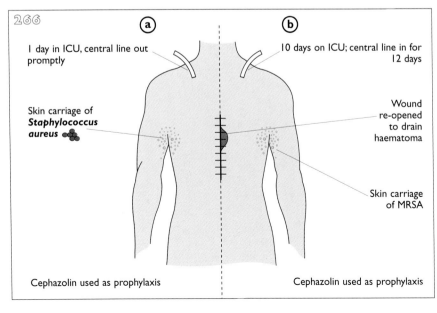

266 Wound infection is less likely to occur in patient (**a**) than in patient (**b**). (ICU: intensive care unit; MRSA: methicillin resistant *Staphylococcus aureus*.)

Infection control in the hospital

Wound infections are part of the spectrum of infections that can be acquired in hospital. The relative incidence of these infections is shown in **267**. UTI are common and arise in many instances from catheterization of the bladder. HAP is also important, and is commoner in the older surgical patient. COAD, compromise of the cough reflex after an abdominal operation, and aspiration of organisms, all increase the likelihood of pneumonia. In the hospital environment antibiotic resistant bacteria are more common, reflecting their selection by the widespread use of antibiotics.

The control of infection in the hospital is integral to the functioning of all aspects of the institution. In the care of patients, good practice of infection control by all health care workers is essential in minimizing the risk of hospital acquired infection. In addition to the wards and outpatient departments, infection control should influence good practice in operating theatres, in sterile instrument supply departments, in the disposal of clinical waste, cleaning services, and hospital catering services.

Different organisms highlight the variety of problems that need to be addressed and these are shown in **268** and **269**. In addition to MRSA, other antibiotic resistant bacteria need to be considered. These include gram-negative organisms such as klebsiella, which can produce a plasmid coded ESBL, or isolates of enterobacter and citrobacter which produce chromosomal coded β-lactamases. The enzymes make these bacteria resistant to a

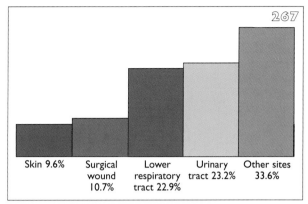

267 Most hospital acquired infections arise in the urinary and respiratory tracts and in surgical wounds.

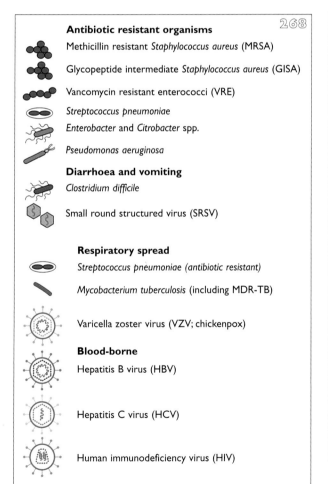

268 Some of the important organisms to consider in hospital acquired infections.

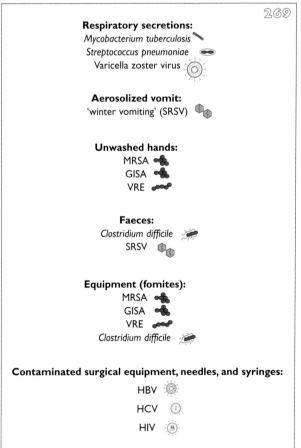

269 Some of the mechanisms whereby hospital acquired infections are spread. (GISA: glycopeptide intermediate *Staphylococcus aureus*; HBV: hepatitis B virus; HCV: hepatitis C virus; HIV: human immunodeficiency virus; MRSA: methicillin resistant *Staphylococcus areus*; SRSV: small round structured virus; VRE: vancomycin resistant enterococcus.)

wide range of β-lactam antibiotics, including most of the cephalosporins. The bacteria can be selected out on a unit by the overuse of one antibiotic, for example cefotaxime. In high care departments such as special baby care units, invasive disease by the gram-negative bacteria cited above can be a problem. The unit may have to be closed to further admissions, alternative antibiotics such as a carbapenem used, and scrupulous infection control practices instituted in order to control the situation.

Diarrhoea can be a major problem in the hospital setting, and *Clostridium difficile* always needs to be considered. In winter, the small round structured viruses (SRSVs) are a particular problem. Aerosolized vomit from an infected patient can contain high concentrations of virus. When this is inhaled and swallowed by other patients, staff, and visitors, they may develop the illness. On open-plan wards there is little that can be done to prevent transmission, and closure of the ward to new admissions, increased cleaning, and minimizing the number of visitors until the 'outbreak' is over, are usually the only options.

Organisms that are spread by the respiratory route include TB, antibiotic resistant pneumococcus, and VZV. A doctor who develops the rash of chickenpox may have infected susceptible mothers on a maternity unit or immuno-compromised patients on a haematology ward. VZV can damage a fetus in the first trimester, produce severe illness in newborns and in pregnant women, as well as life-threatening disseminated illness in susceptible immuno-compromised individuals. Such a scenario means that 'at risk' contacts need their VZV IgG antibody status determined, and susceptible contacts (IgG-negative) need to be given VZV immunoglobulin (VZIG), as passive immunity, in order to reduce their chance of developing the infection.

Blood-borne viruses

HBV, HCV, and HIV are important entities to consider in infection control both in hospital and the community. The patient who may be infected with one or more of these agents poses a risk to health care workers. All 'sharps' injuries, or other incidents where the health care worker comes into contact with blood or body fluid need to be assessed promptly. Washing the affected site with copious amounts of running water is the first step. At the occupational health department or hospital admissions unit, the injured health care worker needs to be advised about further actions to be taken. If the 'donor' is known or considered likely to be HIV-positive, the health care worker is advised to start HIV antiviral post-exposure prophylaxis (PEP) immediately. The risk of HIV in the 'donor' patient can be assessed with information on intravenous drug use, country of origin where HIV prevalence is high, and 'high risk' sexual activities. With the patient's consent, and following appropriate counselling, blood can be taken for serological testing.

In the case of HBV, most health care workers will be vaccinated and protected. Those health care workers who have not responded to the HBV vaccine and who are exposed to an infected patient would be given HBV immunoglobulin (HBIG), which would confer short-term passive immunity. In the case of HCV, PEP regimes are under consideration. It is worthwhile to note that the transmission rate in a significant 'sharps' injury is in the order of 30%, 3% and 0.3% for HBV, HCV, and HIV, respectively.

Health care workers infected with blood-borne viruses also pose a risk to patients. The health care worker who does not respond to the HBV vaccine needs to be counselled to have further blood tests to determine if he or she is a chronic carrier of the virus. Chronic carriage of HBV will exclude the health care worker from performing exposure-prone procedures (EPP) if they are 'high risk' (sAg-positive, eAg-positive, eAb-negative). 'Low risk' carriers, (sAg-positive, eAg-negative, eAb-positive) must have the viral load in blood determined by PCR. If this is over 10^3 genome equivalents/mL, they are also excluded from performing EPP, until successfully treated.

Infection control committee

The infection control committee (ICC) and the infection control team (ICT) coordinate the control of infection within a hospital (**270**). The ICT consists of one or more infection control nurses (ICN) and the infection control doctor (ICD), who is usually a consultant in medical microbiology. They are responsible for the development and implementation of policies and guidelines in the infection control manual. This document is held on all wards and other clinical areas such as outpatient departments, in pathology laboratories, and in hospital operating theatres. The manual should be referred to when a particular problem arises, ranging from a case of open TB or an outbreak of diarrhoea on a ward.

Ongoing awareness and practice of infection control at ward level is done by the link nurses. These ward nurses have an interest in infection control, and are an essential part of the infection control process. Training of these nurses and other hospital staff, as well as audit, are an essential part of the work of the ICN. The ICT reports every 4 months to the ICC, whose membership includes an appropriate range of hospital and community health care workers. In addition to the community ICN, who is the hospital link to nursing homes in the community, the CCDC is important in coordinating infection control issues between the hospital and the community. Managerially the ICC reports to the Trust board, highlighting the role that infection control should have within a hospital.

One important function of the ICT is to identify and act on 'outbreaks' or incidents of infection in the hospital. An outbreak may be defined as two or more cases of a particular infection in one area, for example two cases of MRSA wound infection on an ICU. If the number of cases increases further, the outbreak may be deemed to require the input of all members of the ICC. Here emergency meetings of the ICC may consider it necessary to close the ward to new admissions, increase ward cleaning, and ensure that best practice infection control procedures are in place. Antibiotic use also has to be reviewed, to ensure that particular agents are not used in excess, thus selecting out the resistant organism.

Universal precautions

The control of infection in hospitals is based on a clean working environment, good ward design and facilities, and a good nursing staff to patient ratio (**271a, b**).

270 The composition and functions of the Infection Control Committee and Team.

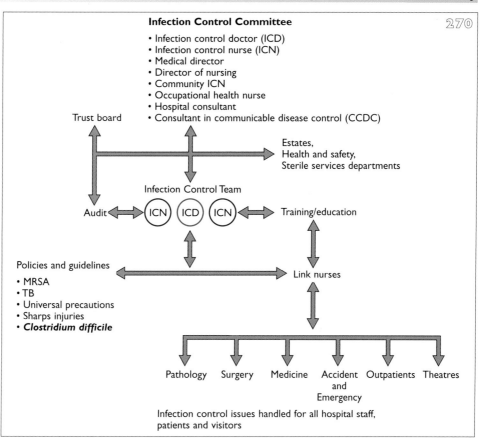

Infection Control Committee

- Infection control doctor (ICD)
- Infection control nurse (ICN)
- Medical director
- Director of nursing
- Community ICN
- Occupational health nurse
- Hospital consultant
- Consultant in communicable disease control (CCDC)

Trust board

Estates, Health and safety, Sterile services departments

Infection Control Team

Audit — ICN — ICD — ICN — Training/education

Policies and guidelines
- MRSA
- TB
- Universal precautions
- Sharps injuries
- *Clostridium difficile*

Link nurses

Pathology   Surgery   Medicine   Accident and Emergency   Outpatients   Theatres

Infection control issues handled for all hospital staff, patients and visitors

271 (**a**) Bad and (**b**) good infection control practice at ward level.

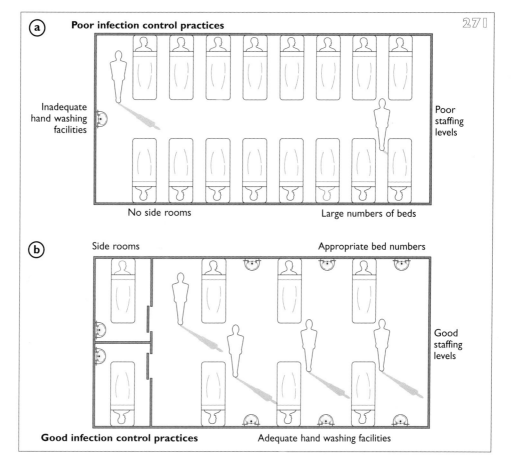

(**a**) **Poor infection control practices**

Inadequate hand washing facilities

Poor staffing levels

No side rooms

Large numbers of beds

(**b**) Side rooms

Appropriate bed numbers

Good staffing levels

Good infection control practices

Adequate hand washing facilities

Every health care worker must make a contribution by adhering to the practice of universal precautions (**272**). Hand washing is such a basic practice and has clearly been shown to reduce the rate of hospital acquired infection. However, health care workers, particularly medical staff, often remain resistant to good practice.

Risk assessment in infection control

An example of risk assessment in infection control, and good and bad practice is shown in **273a, b**. A patient is admitted to hospital with a gastrointestinal bleed. The admitting doctor notes that the patient has a cough and promptly reviews a chest X-ray, which indicates that TB is a possibility; a ZN stain shows AFB. The patient is nursed in a side room according to infection control practice. Bad practice is where the cough is ignored, a chest X-ray is done but not reviewed and the patient is placed on the open ward. Days later the diagnosis of TB is considered and then confirmed. By this time other patients, staff, and visitors have been exposed. Contact tracing needs to be done to identify patients and staff who are at risk. As with all infection control situations such as this, the work involved is time consuming.

Until recently it was generally accepted that the use of reusable surgical equipment did not pose a health risk. Providing surgical equipment was adequately washed, decontaminated/disinfected and then sterilized, it was considered safe to use on all other patients. Decontamination and disinfection are processes that remove all vegetative bacteria. Sterilization is the process that destroys all organisms, including bacterial spores. Standard sterilization of equipment in a hospital usually employs a vacuum and steam autoclave working at 135°C for 3 minutes.

The transmissible spongiform encephalopathies (TSEs)

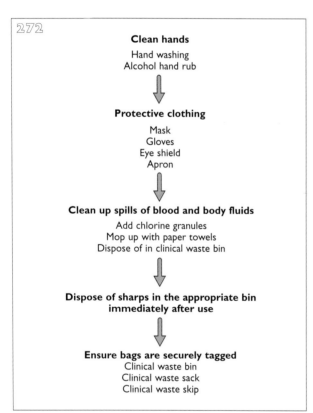

272 Universal precautions: clean hands, wearing protective clothing, cleaning up blood spills, safe disposal of sharps, correct disposal of clinical waste.

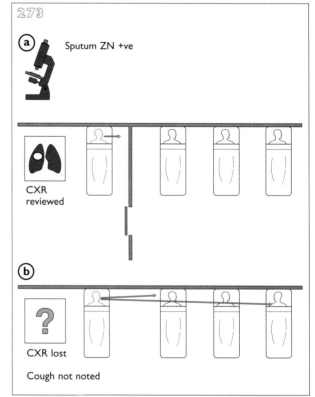

273 Good and bad practice in risk assessment of a patient with tuberculosis. (**a**) Prompt review of the chest X-ray (CXR) and a positive microscopy result means that the patient is admitted to a side room. (**b**) When tuberculosis is not considered, the infectious patient on the open ward poses a risk to other patients.

have dramatically influenced the situation in recent years. The appearance of variant Creutzfeltd-Jakob disease (vCJD) following the bovine spongiform encephalopathy crisis (BSE) in cattle in the United Kingdom is the main reason. The TSEs are a group of transmissible proteinaceous agents termed prions, which cause progressive neurological degeneration, for which there is no cure. Familial and sporadic cases of disease associated with these agents have been recognized for decades. In the 1980s their importance as transmissible agents was shown when individuals, who had received natural human growth hormone harvested from cadavers, developed CJD. Amongst the cadaveric pituitary glands were some from individuals who had died of CJD. The use of natural hormone was banned in 1985, and only synthetic hormone was allowed. Similarly some individuals who received human dura mater grafts have also developed CJD.

The problem with TSEs is that they are resistant to the standard methods of sterilization. This means that when a patient with a TSE undergoes an invasive procedure, there is no guarantee that the surgical instruments used will be free of the agent before they are used in the next patient. The problem is exacerbated by the fact that CJD or related neurological conditions may only be considered weeks or months after a patient has undergone an invasive procedure, by which time the equipment may have been used on many other individuals.

Risk assessment should thus become part of standard clinical care. An example of risk assessment for TSE is shown in **274**. Such a document should be used when a patient gives consent for an invasive procedure where reusable surgical equipment is to be used. The usefulness of such an assessment at the earliest stage of a hospital stay is obvious.

274

All patients who are undergoing a surgical procedure should be asked the following questions. If they answer 'yes' to any of these questions, you must contact a member of the infection control team NOW before any invasive procedure is started.

Has the patient ever received natural human growth hormone?*	Y	N
Has the patient ever received any other natural human pituitary hormone?*	Y	N
Is there a family history of CJD or a related condition?** (includes parent, grandparent, grandchild, brother, sister)	Y	N
Has the patient had any neurological or ENT procedure before 1993, where a human dura mater graft was used?	Y	N

The clinical team must provide the answer to the following question:

Is CJD or other related condition part of the differential diagnosis?	Y	N

* This relates only to hormones that were harvested from the pituitary gland of human cadavers, a practice discontinued in 1985

** In addition to CJD, variant CJD, Gertsman-Straussler syndrome and Fatal Familial Insomnia are related conditions

274 A risk assessment document for Creutzfeltd-Jakob disease (CJD) and related conditions. (ENT: ear, nose, and throat.)

Infection control in the community

Infections in the community can have a range of implications. As outlined in **275a–c**, a particular infection in one person can have a number of consequences. For a 23-year-old female office worker with an uncomplicated UTI there will be no public health implications. If the same person develops meningococcal meningitis, contacts of that person need to be identified by the CCDC or public health doctor and offered prophylactic antibiotics and vaccination. The aim of the antibiotic is not to lessen the chance of an individual developing meningococcal infection, but to reduce the carriage rate of the organism in a cohort of people. If the same 23-year-old worked in a 'fast food' outlet and developed diarrhoea, with

Escherichia coli O157 being isolated from her stool, there would be a wider range of public health issues. As asymptomatic infection can occur, family members and the other 'fast food' employees would have to be screened for the organism. A detailed review of the food preparation in the shop would have to be conducted by Environmental Health Officers (EHOs) and selected food samples collected for microbiological testing. GPs in the area would need to be alerted about the problem.

Outbreaks at the local and national level

The extent that a particular organism is a problem in the community is shown as an 'iceberg' in **276**. A small proportion of infected individuals may be symptomatic. Some

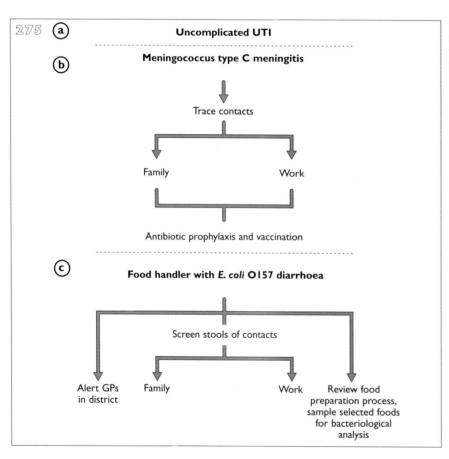

275 Infection in the community can have different implications. (**a**) Urinary tract infection (UTI); (**b**) meningococcal C infection; (**c**) *Escherichia coli* O157.

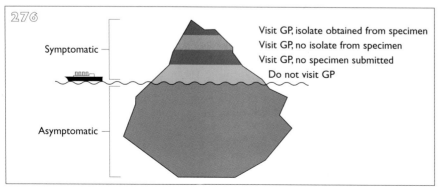

276 The 'iceberg' shows that an organism can exist in the community at various levels.

of these visit their GP, of whom a number submit a specimen, and the organism is isolated from a few of these specimens. It is from this final group that the identity of the agent causing the problem in the community is made. However, as many individuals have asymptomatic infection they will provide the reservoir of the organism. STI such as chlamydia is an example where the majority of infected individuals have no symptoms.

The information on isolates obtained in microbiology laboratories is essential for local, regional and national surveillance. The number of organisms identified each week by one laboratory may be small, but if this information is collated at regional level, useful pictures can be produced. Using data from the West Midlands of the United Kingdom, combined weekly updates of laboratory reports of important community infection control problems can be made (**277a–c**). RSV infection is a winter illness and not surprisingly distinct peaks of activity occur in this period each year. Campylobacter has an unacceptably high rate throughout the year, reflecting the ubiquitous nature of the organism. On the other hand, *Salmonella typhimurium* is uncommon, but in late summer of 2000 the collated regional data identified an outbreak associated with this organism. The information was used by the regional CCDC to identify a source, which was found to be contaminated salad being brought into the region, which was used in the preparation of 'fast food'.

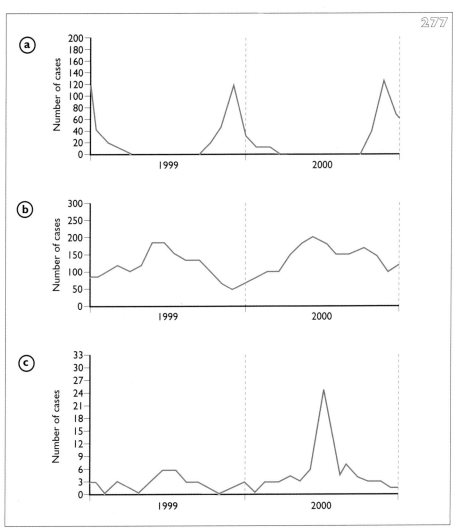

277 The pattern of weekly reporting of data in 1999 and 2000 from the West Midlands of the United Kingdom. (**a**) Respiratory syncitial virus; (**b**) campylobacter; (**c**) *Salmonella typhimurium*.

It is important once an outbreak has been identified that the source of the offending agent is identified in order to prevent recurrences. Consider 22 individuals out of 50 who developed diarrhoea and vomiting after eating 'take away' food at a school fair. From 5 of these individuals salmonella was isolated from stool specimens. A graph showing the time that symptoms started after the fair (+/- 2 days), would be compatible with a single source of the organism, identified here as *Salmonella enteriditis* (**278a**). The offending food can be identified by risk assessment. Assume that only two types of food were available at the fair, hamburger and chicken mayonnaise roll. The food history of all 50 individuals is taken and collated, and an attack rate calculated (**278b**). This clearly shows that the chicken mayonnaise roll is the offending food, as the attack rate is 80% compared to 8% in those who ate the hamburger. Ideally the attack rates should be 100% and 0% respectively. However, the two ill individuals who ate hamburgers may have had a small portion of chicken roll from someone else, or they may have had symptoms for other reasons. Closer investigation reveals that the travelling 'take away' owner prepares his own mayonnaise using raw eggs contaminated with salmonella. As the mayonnaise is kept at room temperature, it delivers salmonella to all those who consume the chicken mayonnaise rolls at fairs where the 'take away' goes! Clearly the EHO would put a stop to this.

National reporting

Communication of information about infectious diseases must also be done at national level, for it is only by national reporting that an international problem can be identified. Consider five cases of legionella pneumonia occurring in five separate cities over a 6-week period (**279a**). At the local level each microbiologist and CCDC may be aware that an individual had been on holiday in an island resort several days before the illness developed. On its own this information is useless, but if countrywide data is collected by a national body such as the Communicable Diseases Surveillance Centre, London, or the Center for Disease Control, Atlanta, USA, it is possible to recognize that an outbreak may be in progress (**279b**). Information from all five affected individuals will show that during their holiday they all stayed at the same hotel and used the same jacuzzi. The local authorities for the resort would be informed, and they must then investigate the likely source of legionella and ensure that it is not used until it is made safe.

Notification of infectious diseases

It is very important that certain infectious diseases are reported to the local public health doctor or CCDC as soon as a diagnosis has been made. This is done so that contacts of a case, for example of meningococcal sepsis, can be identified and given antibiotic prophylaxis. In many instances a clinical diagnosis may be confirmed promptly in the laboratory by the isolation of the particular organism. However, clinical diagnosis alone is also important. Several patients suffering from 'food poisoning' may attend different GPs in an area; none of these patients may submit a stool specimen for examination, or if they do, an organism may not be identified. However, if all the GPs concerned inform the CCDC of their cases of food poisoning, it would be possible to build up a picture of a single source for an outbreak. In conjunction with the EHO of the area, an investigation of food outlets may identify an infected food handler, and/or contaminated food.

It is a statutory requirement of every clinician attending a patient who is suffering from one of the diseases listed below to notify the public health doctors or CCDC at the earliest opportunity. The list of notifiable diseases is listed in the Public Health (Infectious Diseases) Regulations of 1988 based on an Act of Parliament of 1984. The list of notifiable diseases for England and Wales is shown below. Unfortunately this list is somewhat outdated and significant omissions exist such as legionella and the water-borne parasite cryptosporidium.

- Acute encephalitis
- Acute poliomyelitis
- Anthrax
- Cholera
- Diphtheria
- Dysentery
- Food poisoning (including suspected food poisoning)
- Lassa fever
- Leprosy
- Leptospirosis
- Malaria
- Measles
- Meninigitis
- Meningococcal septicaemia (without meningitis)
- Mumps
- Ophthalmia neonatorum
- Paratyphoid fever
- Plague (*Yersinia pestis*)
- Rabies
- Relapsing fever
- Rubella
- Scarlet fever (group A streptococcus)
- Smallpox
- Tetanus
- Tuberculosis (all forms)
- Typhoid fever
- Typhus
- Viral haemorrhagic fever (for example Ebola, Rift Valley Fever)
- Viral hepatitis (A, B, C)
- Whooping cough
- Yellow fever

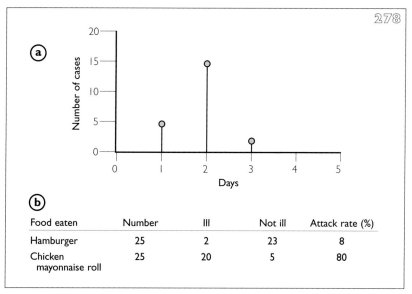

278 (a) Plotting the time after food consumption to symptoms of disease identifies a single source for the outbreak. **(b)** A food history enables the attack rate to be determined, so that offending food can be identified.

Food eaten	Number	Ill	Not ill	Attack rate (%)
Hamburger	25	2	23	8
Chicken mayonnaise roll	25	20	5	80

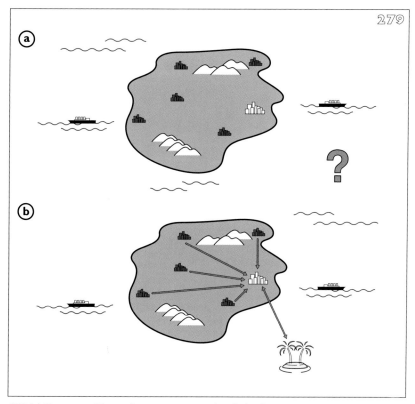

279 (a) Five cases of legionella pneumonia are identified in five separate cities in a country. **(b)** Only if all the cases are referred to a central surveillance unit, will it be possible to recognize an international problem.

International travel

International travel is a major industry nowadays, and it is not surprising that it carries a risk of infection. The examples are many and range from common conditions such as food poisoning to the more uncommon legionellosis. Taking a travel history from the patient and discussing this with the medical microbiologist will determine which investigations need to be done. For example, a young man who has returned from a holiday visiting relatives in the Indian subcontinent and who is complaining of headache, fever, and malaise should be investigated for malaria (blood smears) and typhoid (blood culture) in the first instance. An outline of the main risks and the precautions to take when travelling are shown in **280a–c**, and can be summarized as food, drink, malaria, and sex.

An 'eco challenge' race in Borneo in 2000 involved 312 athletes from 26 countries undertaking a gruelling trip through forests and rivers. Half of the participants acquired leptospirosis from the event.

Vaccination

Immunity to infection can be classed as passive or active.

Passive immunity

Maternal IgG antibodies cross the placenta in the later stages of a normal pregnancy and protect the child against a wide range of infections for several months. Passive immunity can also be given by using hyperimmune globulin (IG). Although the effect is short term, susceptible individuals who have been exposed to either HBV or VZV can be protected by HBIG and VZIG. Newborns whose mothers are 'high risk' carriers of HBV are vaccinated with the HBV vaccine and given HBIG, obtained from individuals with natural immunity to HBV. Similarly, non-immune individuals at risk of serious chickenpox infection, such as those who are pregnant, newborn, or immunocompromised are given VZIG. The problem with passive immunity is demonstrated by the fact that VZIG may fail to protect about 50% of those who receive it.

Active immunity

Active immunity has been practised since the time of Jenner, who in 1790 showed that vaccination with cowpox virus could protect individuals from the more virulent smallpox virus. It was in the twentieth century that vaccination triumphed and it is now an essential aspect of human health. Advances in science, exemplified by virus production in cell culture, virus purification, and genetic engineering, have enabled a wide range of effective vaccines to be produced.

An outline of various vaccines is shown in **281**. Vaccines can be grouped into live, killed, toxoid, and conjugated. Live viral vaccines are obtained by multiple passage of a virus in cell culture. This results in attenuation of the virulence of the virus, but its antigenic properties are maintained. When a live vaccine is given, the virus replicates at a low level, and an efficient immune response is mounted. Immunocompromised individuals should not

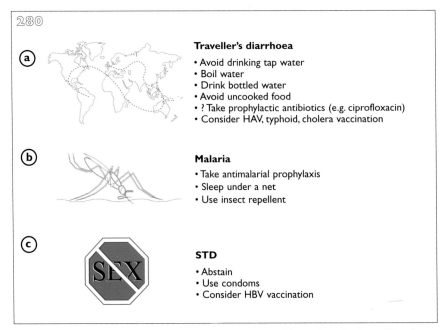

Traveller's diarrhoea
- Avoid drinking tap water
- Boil water
- Drink bottled water
- Avoid uncooked food
- ? Take prophylactic antibiotics (e.g. ciprofloxacin)
- Consider HAV, typhoid, cholera vaccination

Malaria
- Take antimalarial prophylaxis
- Sleep under a net
- Use insect repellent

STD
- Abstain
- Use condoms
- Consider HBV vaccination

280 Some health advice for the international traveller. Avoiding: (**a**) travellers diarrhoea; (**b**) malaria; (**c**) sexually transmitted disease (STD).

An intact microbe can cause its disease

Disease — IgG
— IgA
Secretory IgA is protective in mucosal secretions
IgM
Stimulates potent immune response which can be protective for life

An attenuated vaccine contains microbes that replicate in host tissues but do not usually cause disease, e.g. polio live vaccine. Disease can occur in immunocompromised individuals (e.g. AIDS patients). [Polio, MMR, typhoid]

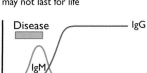

No disease — IgG
— IgA
Secretory IgA is protective in bowel secretions
IgM
Stimulates potent immune response including IgA

An inactivated killed vaccine contains microbes that are unable to replicate. Safe to use in all patients. [Polio, HAV, cholera]

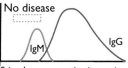

No disease   IgG
IgM   IgA
Stimulates proctective immunity which may not last for life

A toxin such as tetanus toxin is active, i.e. causes disease and is immunogenic

Disease — IgG
IgM
Stimulates protective immunity which can be active for life

A toxoid (e.g. tetanus) used in vaccination is inactive but is still immunogenic. Formalin is used for inactivation. [Diphtheria, pertussis, tetanus]

No disease
IgM   IgG
Stimulates protective immunity which may not last for life

Immunity to the PRP capsule of *Haemophilus influenzae* is T cell- independent, and the immune response is poor

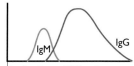

Poor immune response to T-cell indepentant antigen

PRP conjugated to tetanus toxoid is converted to a T cell-dependent antigen and is immunogenic as a conjugated vaccine. [Hib]

IgM   IgG
Antibodies to PRP and tetanus toxin

281 The principles of vaccination.

be given live vaccines, as these attenuated viruses cannot be controlled, and overwhelming infection may occur.

With 'killed' vaccines, the organism is inactivated by chemical treatment such as formalin, but its antigenicity is maintained. As there is no reproduction of the organism, the number of cells recruited to the site of the injection is low. The immune memory is not as marked as that with a live vaccine and antibody levels may wane over years. Toxoids are bacterial toxins that have also been inactivated, but maintain their immunogenicity. Conjugated vaccines are those where the antigen has been linked to another molecule; an example is the Hib vaccine. The PrP component of *Haemophilus influenzae* serotype b is not immunogenic on its own. However, when linked to a protein carrier, such as the tetanus toxoid, it becomes T cell dependent and antibodies are produced to it, as well as the tetanus toxoid.

The vaccination program for children in the United Kingdom is shown in **282**. Many other vaccines are available and include influenza and pneumococcal vaccine, recommended for individuals over 65 years of age or those with chronic heart and lung disease. HBV vaccine has been essential in protecting health care workers. Hepatitis A virus, typhoid, and cholera vaccines are available for travellers. The global effectiveness of vaccines is exemplified by the fact that smallpox has been eliminated throughout the world, and polio should be eliminated in the first years of the twentyfirst century.

Comment

The following references highlight some of the important aspects of infection control both in hospital and the community:

Donksey CJ, Chowdhry TK, Hecker MT *et al.* (2000). Effect of antibiotic therapy on the density of vancomycin resistant enterococci in the stool of colonised patients. *New England Journal of Medicine* 343: 1925–32.

Foca M, Jakob K, Whittier S *et al.* (2000). Endemic *Pseudomonas aeruginosa* infection in a neonatal intensive care unit. *New England Journal of Medicine* 343: 695–700.

Ross RS, Viazov S, Gross T, Hofmann F, Seipp H-M, Roggendorf M (2000). Transmission of hepatitis C virus from patient to an anesthesiology assistant to five patients. *New England Journal of Medicine* 343: 1851–4.

Ryan ET, Kain KC (2000). Health advice and immunisation for travellers. *New England Journal of Medicine* 343: 1716–24.

Whitney CG, Farley MM, Hadler J *et al.* (2000). Increased prevalence of multi-drug resistant *Streptococcus pneumoniae* in the United States. *New England Journal of Medicine* 343: 1917–24. (Also see editorial comment, pp. 1961–3.)

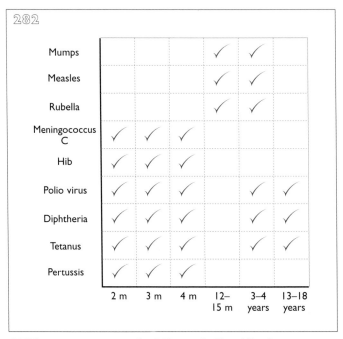

282 The vaccination program for children in the United Kingdom. (Hib: *Haemophilus influenzae* b.)

Index